English

for Medical Assistants

Kommunikation mit Patienten in der Arztpraxis
Verwaltung • Diagnose • Therapie

von Silke Gerdes

Holland + Josenhans/Handwerk und Technik

Bildquellenverzeichnis

Zeichnungen, soweit nicht anders angegeben: Gabriele Timm, Kaarst

adpic Bildagentur, Bonn: S.22, 52 b, 73, 74, 80, 104, 121; AOK Mediendienst: S. 15, 113, 118 b; Beckman Coulter GmbH, Krefeld: S. 99; DHD Multimedia Gallery, Damon Hart-Davis: S. 93; Herb Allgaier, Stuttgart: S. 40b; Silke Gerdes, Hamburg: 119 a, 129 b; SUAVA Pressedienst, Luzern: S.139; Verlag Handwerk und Technik, Hamburg (HT 4580): S.33 (3M Deutschland GmbH, Neuss), 76 a; Verlag Holland + Josenhans, Stuttgart: (H+J 5897): S. 11, 52 a, (H+J 5820): S. 16 a, b, 40 a, 57, 62, 68, 69 g, 76 b, 134; www.fotolia.de: S. 5, 7, 21, 46

ISBN 978-3-7782-1724-5
Schülerausgabe – 2. durchgesehene Auflage 2015

ISBN 978-3-7782-1725-2
Lehrerausgabe mit Lösungen – II/2. Auflage

Verlag Holland+Josenhans GmbH & Co. KG, Postfach 102352, 70019 Stuttgart – 2015
Tel.: 0711/6143920, Fax: 0711/6143922, E-Mail: info@handwerk-technik.de
Internet: www.handwerk-technik.de

Redaktionelle Mitarbeit (Englisch): Melissa Martin
Umschlagabbildungen: www.fotolia.de; adpic Bildagentur, 53121 Bonn
Layout: Oleg Kovalevski, 70563 Stuttgart
Satz: CMS – Cross Media Solutions GmbH, 97080 Würzburg
Druck und Weiterverarbeitung: Konrad Triltsch, Print und digitale Medien GmbH, 97199 Ochsenfurt-Hohestadt

English for Medical Assistants ist ein neues Lehrwerk für die Berufsschule und berufliche Weiterbildung, das speziell für medizinisches Assistenzpersonal entwickelt wurde. Schwerpunkte sind entsprechend die Bereiche Verwaltung, Diagnose und Therapie, in denen Patientenkommunikation auf Englisch stattfindet. Dabei werden sowohl Sprachkenntnisse für die Kommunikation mit Patienten im allgemein-medizinisch-internistischen Bereich als auch mit anderen Fachbereichen vermittelt. Im Berufsschulunterricht der medizinischen Fachangestellten (MFA) bietet sich dieses Lehrwerk zur Vertiefung an.

Ziel von **English for Medical Assistants** ist die angemessene Betreuung englischsprachiger Patienten und Patientinnen im praxisorientierten Dialog. Ein Schwerpunkt des Lehrwerks besteht im Einüben und Anwenden des berufsrelevanten Wortschatzes, ein weiterer in dem Erwerb der Sprachkompetenz durch Übungen zu Hörverständnis, Leseverständnis, Sprechfertigkeit und durch spielerische Übungen. Das jedes Kapitel abschließende Rollenspiel bereitet den Lerner darauf vor, seine Sprachkompetenz am Arbeitsplatz kompetent anzuwenden.

Hilfestellung wird dabei gegeben durch:

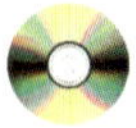

Dialoge auf der Audio-CD: Sie dienen dem motivierenden Einstieg ins jeweilige Thema und schulen das Hörverstehen. Sie bereiten außerdem unterstützend auf die jeweils folgende Dialogübung vor.

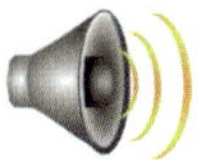

Aussprachehilfe: Medizinische Fachwörter in den Lesetexten, die nicht in den Audio-Dialogen vorkommen, können über die Tracks der Audio-Vokabelhilfe auf der CD angehört und die Aussprache geübt werden.

9 severity – Schweregrad
10 treadmill – Laufband

Vokabelhilfen direkt beim Text erleichtern das Erarbeiten des Inhalts.

Das Lehrwerk wurde für Schüler geschrieben, deren Englischkenntnisse dem Niveau des Sekundarabschlusses 1 entsprechen. Es werden keine Kenntnisse des englischen medizinischen Fachvokabulars vorausgesetzt. Einige Units bieten Aufgaben für leistungsstärkere Schüler (z.B. German Role Cards). Am besten lernt es sich, wenn im Lernfeldunterricht vorher schon ein Thema behandelt wurde (z.B. EKG) und sich der Englischunterricht verknüpfend mit dem entsprechenden Thema befasst.

Da die medizinischen Fachbegriffe in der amerikanischen Variante leichter zu lesen und zu verstehen sind, wird im Buch die amerikanische Schreibweise bevorzugt. Auf Grammatik wird im Buch bewusst verzichtet, da der Schwerpunkt auf der Kommunikation liegt. Die Nutzer sollen zum Gebrauch der englischen Sprache unter Anwendung des Fachvokabulars ermutigt werden.

Der Verlag und die Autorin wünschen bei der Arbeit mit **English for Medical Assistants** viel Erfolg.

Inhalt

1 Guidelines on Healthcare in Germany

1.1 Health Insurance

READING

1 **Read the following text and find the German words 2. Check any other new vocabulary in the vocabulary list or in a dictionary.**

In Germany health insurance is compulsory. You can choose your health insurance company. Normally, employees are covered by a statutory health insurance policy. If their income is above a certain limit employees can also choose a private insurance. If you are unemployed or get social welfare you are covered through the Federal Employment Office.

Statutory health insurance

The monthly insurance contribution depends upon your income. Unemployed spouses, children and young adults under 25 can be co-insured free of charge under the statutory health insurance policy.
Each family member has a personal health insurance card that contains data such as full name, date of birth and insurance number. This card has to be presented at the first doctor's visit every quarter.

Private health insurance

If your income exceeds a certain limit you can also choose to be privately insured. However, family members cannot be co-insured free of charge. Private patients do not have to pay a practice charge. You can also see a specialist without a referral. The doctor sends the bill to the patient. The patient sends it to the health insurance company.

statutory health insurance
vaccination
referral

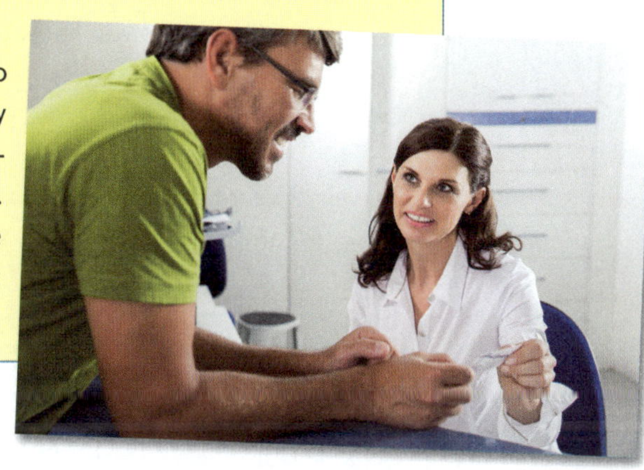

COMPREHENSION

2 **Find the following words in the text:**

gesetzliche Krankenversicherung | verpflichtend | Arbeitnehmer
private Krankenversicherung | Sozialhilfe | Versicherungsbeitrag
abhängen von | Ehepartner | Erwachsene | mitversichert
kostenfrei | Daten | Quartal
ausgenommen | Einkommen | Vorsorgeuntersuchung
Impfungen | überweisen | zusätzlich

3 **Answer the following questions:**

1. What kind of health insurance do most people in Germany have?

   ....

2. Who can have private health insurance?

   ....

3. Who can be co-insured?

   ....

4. What information does a health insurance chip card contain?

   ....

DIALOG

4 *Swavek Pik is a Polish employee who wants to start working in a garage. He is 28 years old and has a wife and a 14 months old son. His family still lives in Poland. Because he does not have health insurance yet, he asks for some information about the health insurance system in Germany:*

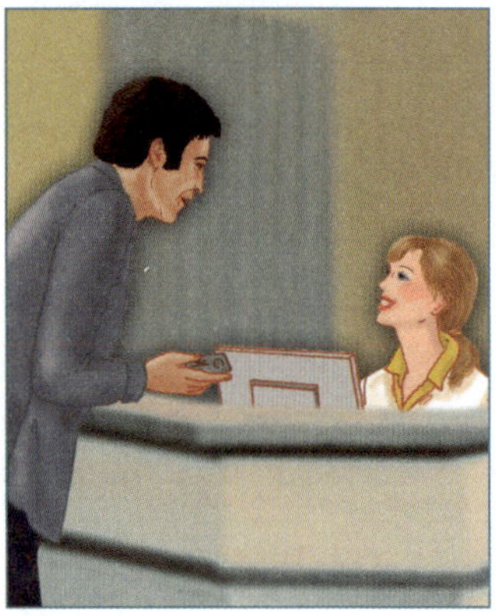

Swavek: I am still looking for a statutory health insurance company. Do you know any?

You: ....

Swavek: I heard that I need a health insurance card. Will the company give me such a card? And what do I need it for?

You: ....

....

....

Swavek: But I do not know much about the German health care system. For example, I have a wife and a small son. Do I have to insure them, too? She has no work at the moment.

You: ....

....

....

....

Swavek: How much insurance contribution do I have to pay?

You: ....

Swavek: Do I have to pay cash after the doctor's visit?

You: ....

1.2 Doctor's Visits

LISTENING Track 1

1 **Listen to the dialog and answer the following questions:**

- *Why is the patient in the doctor's practice?*
- *What information does the medical assistant give?*

BE: Arztpraxis – surgery

READING

2 **Read the following text and find the German words 3. Check any other new vocabulary in the vocabulary list or in a dictionary.**

It is recommended that patients have a family doctor who is normally a general practitioner (GP) or internist. They are familiar with the patient's medical history and, if necessary, can refer him/her to a specialist. Then the GP writes out a referral which the patient has to give to the specialist (e.g. an orthopedic specialist). The referral note only states the type of treatment or tests the patient needs. The patient then chooses the doctor himself or herself.

referral
orthopedic specialist
statutory health insurance

If the patient needs some prescription medication, the doctor will write a prescription which has to be presented at the pharmacist's. Patients who are covered by statutory health insurance normally have to make a co-payment of 5 to 10 euros, depending on the price of the drug.

Some medicines are not covered by the health insurance companies. Then the doctor will write out a private prescription and the patient has to pay the full costs. The same applies for over-the-counter medicine. Minors do not have to pay prescription charges.

If the patient has private health insurance he or she only gets private prescriptions and has to pay the costs of the medicines first. The patient will then send the prescription form to the private health insurance company who will repay the costs.

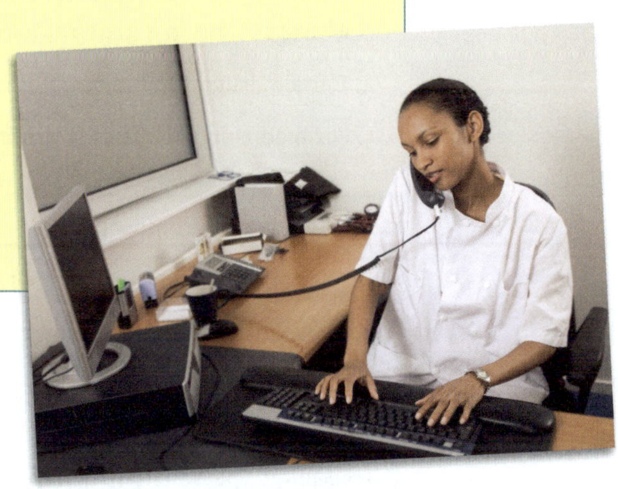

COMPREHENSION

3 Find the following words in the text:

empfehlen · Allgemeinmediziner · Patientenvorgeschichte

überweisen · ärztliche Überweisung · Rezeptgebühr · Orthopäde

rezeptpflichtig · gelten · Apotheker · Zuzahlung

Minderjährige · Medikament · abgedeckt · freiverkäuflich

4 What are these documents called in English?

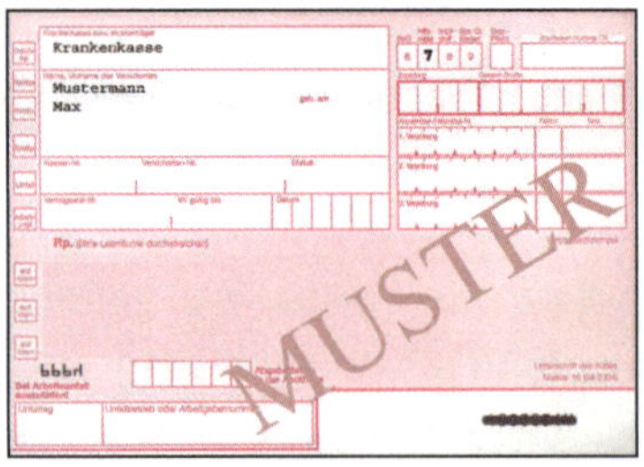

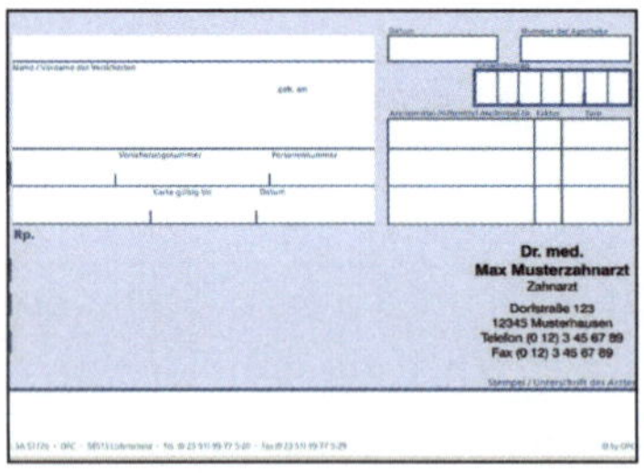

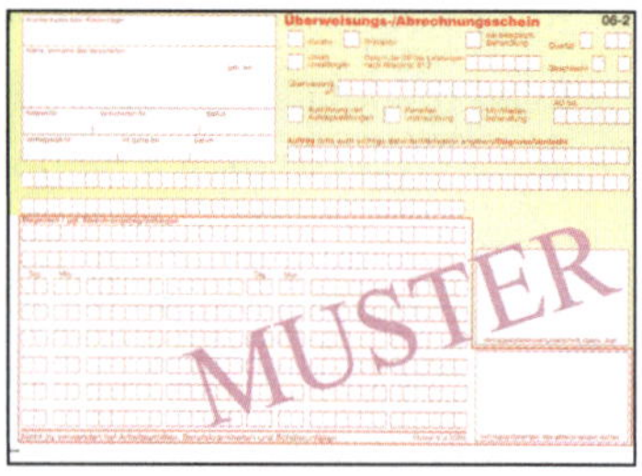

5 Match the sentence parts:

1. It is good to have a family doctor	a. you can choose the specialist yourself.
2. When you need to see a medical specialist	b. you need a private prescription.
3. When you have a referral for a doctor who specilizes in e.g. dermatology	c. are called over-the counter medicines.
4. Certain drugs such as antibiotics	d. the patient has to pay the full price.
5. For medicines on the pink prescription	e. because s/he knows the patient's medical history.
6. For the contraceptive pill	f. do not have to pay prescription charges.
7. For medicines on the blue prescription	g. you should have a referral from your GP.
8. The statutory heath insurance	h. you have to make co-payments.
9. Medicines which you can buy without having a prescription	i. does not cover the costs of private prescriptions.
10. Minors (persons under 18 years)	j. you get only on prescription.

DIALOG / ROLEPLAY

6 **With a partner write a dialog. Complete the speech bubbles:**

Rick Raymond from South Africa married a German woman and moved to Germany five months ago. This morning he got a terrible lumbago and decided to see his GP Dr. Rose. She wrote him a referral to see an orthopedist. The medical assistant has given him a pink and a blue prescription. Rick Raymond is looking very confused.

MFA bietet Patient ihre Hilfe an:

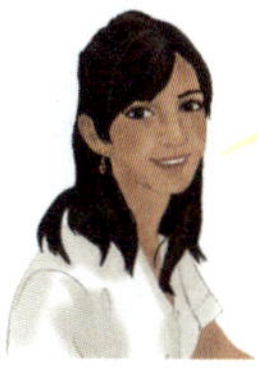

....

Zunächst möchte Mr. Raymond etwas über das Formular der Ärztin wissen.

....

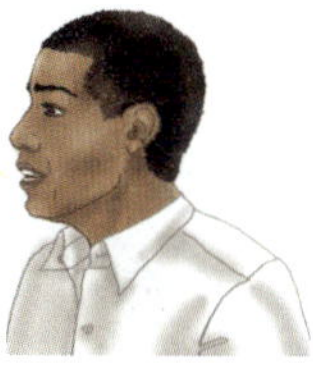

MFA erklärt, was Patient mit dem Überweisungsschein machen muss:

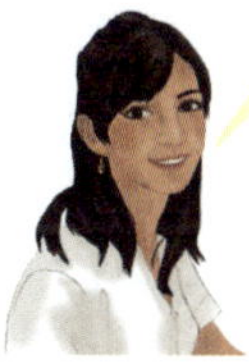

....

....

....

....

....

Mr. Raymond fragt, ob auch Name und Adresse des Orthopäden auf der Überweisung steht:

....

....

....

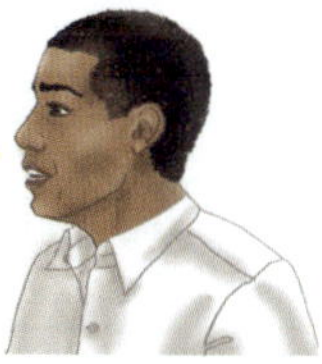

MFA antwortet:

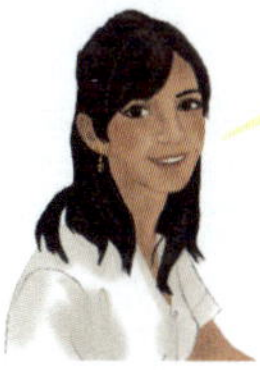

....

Patient versteht und fragt jetzt, was es mit den anderen zwei Formularen auf sich hat:

....

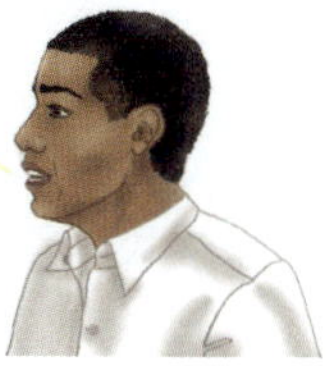

MFA sagt, dass es sich um Rezepte handelt, die der Patient in der Apotheke vorlegen muss. Er benötigt die Rezepte, da die Medikamente verschreibungspflichtig sind.

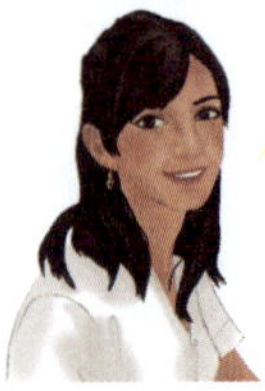

Patient fragt, warum es unterschiedliche Farben sind:

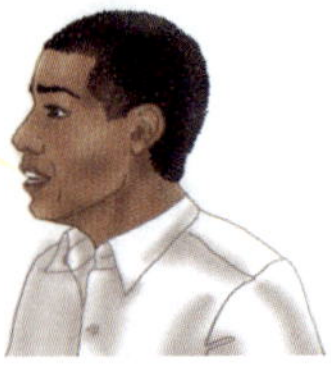

MFA nennt die Unterschiede der Rezepte.

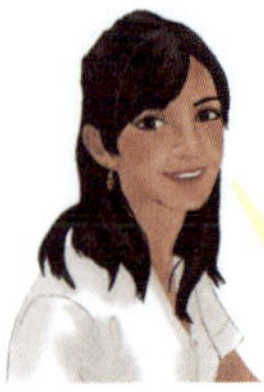

Patient bedankt sich für die Erklärungen und fragt noch nach einem Orthopäden in der Nähe. Er wohnt in der Danziger Straße in 20099 Hamburg.

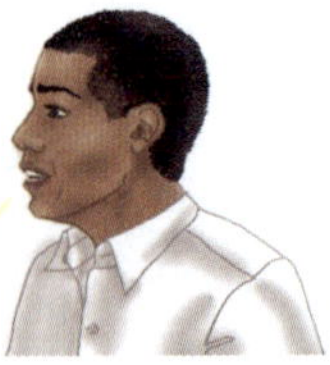

MFA schaut im Handbuch nach und schlägt dem Patient zwei Orthopäden mit Adresse vor.

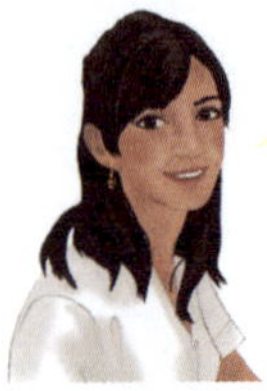

Patient entscheidet sich für den 2. Vorschlag, weil es näher ist.

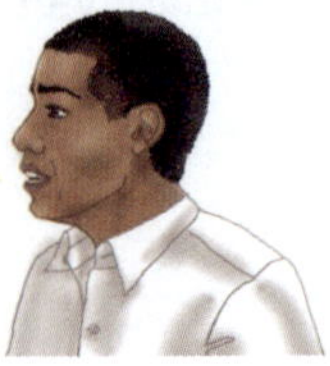

Sie gibt ihm eine Notiz mit der Anschrift, Telefonnummer und Sprechzeiten des Arztes, wünscht ihm gute Besserung und verabschiedet sich.

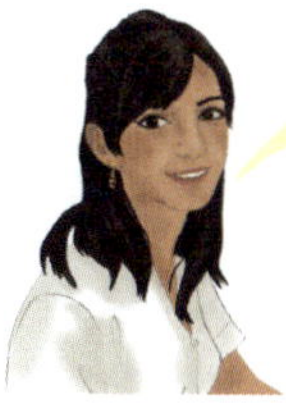

Patient bedankt sich nochmals und verabschiedet sich.

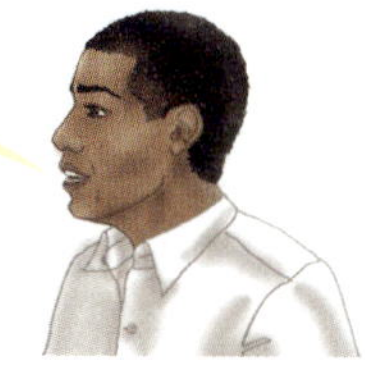

1.3 Sick Leave

LISTENING 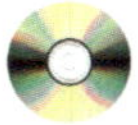 Track 2

1 **Listen to the dialog and answer the following questions:**

- *Why is the patient in the doctor's practice?*
- *What information does the medical assistant give?*

READING

2 **Read the following text and find the German words 3. Check any other new vocabulary in the vocabulary list or in a dictionary.**

Employees who are ill have to inform their employer. After the third day of illness they need a doctor's certificate, a so called sick note. It states the dates of the beginning and the expected end of the temporary illness. The certificate includes three forms – one must be given to the employer, one to the health insurance company and one stays at the doctor's. The form for the employer does not include the diagnosis, the form for the insurance company does.

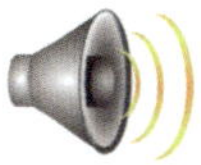

diagnosis

COMPREHENSION

3 **Find the following words in the text:**

Arbeitnehmer | Arbeitgeber | ärztliche Bescheinigung | Krankschreibung | angeben/nennen | zeitliche Arbeitsunfähigkeit | Formular | Krankenversicherung | Diagnose

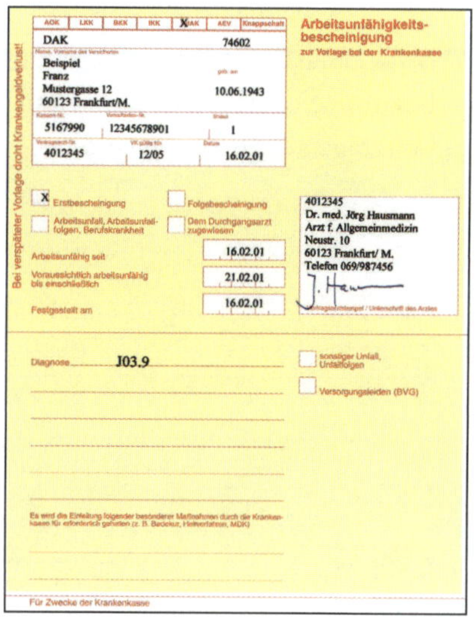

Arbeitsunfähigkeits-bescheinigung
zur Vorlage bei der Krankenkasse

AOK | LKK | BKK | IKK | X DAK | AEV | Knappschaft

DAK 74602
Beispiel
Franz
Mustergasse 12
60123 Frankfurt/M.
geb. am 10.06.1943
5167990 12345678901 1
4012345 12/05 16.02.01

Bei verspäteter Vorlage droht Krankengeldverlust!

X Erstbescheinigung
Folgebescheinigung
Arbeitsunfall, Arbeitsunfallfolgen, Berufskrankheit
Dem Durchgangsarzt zugewiesen
Arbeitsunfähig seit 16.02.01
Voraussichtlich arbeitsunfähig bis einschließlich 21.02.01
Festgestellt am 16.02.01

4012345
Dr. med. Jörg Hausmann
Arzt f. Allgemeinmedizin
Neustr. 10
60123 Frankfurt/ M.
Telefon 069/987456
Vertragsarztstempel / Unterschrift des Arztes

Diagnose J03.9
sonstiger Unfall, Unfallfolgen
Versorgungsleiden (BVG)

Es wird die Einleitung folgender besonderer Maßnahmen durch die Krankenkasse für erforderlich gehalten (z. B. Badekur, Heilverfahren, MDK)

Für Zwecke der Krankenkasse

4 **Answer the following questions:**

1. When do employees have to give a sick note to their employers?

2. What information can you find on the sick note?

3. True or false?: The sick note must be sent to the health insurance.

DIALOG / ROLEPLAY

5 **With a partner write a dialog. Complete the speech bubbles:**

Padmé Khan, a 27 year old patient from India who works for an IT company, comes out of the treatment room with a sick note. She is looking confused. She does not know what she has to do with it. The medical assistant is offering her help.

MFA fragt Patientin, ob sie Hilfe benötigt.

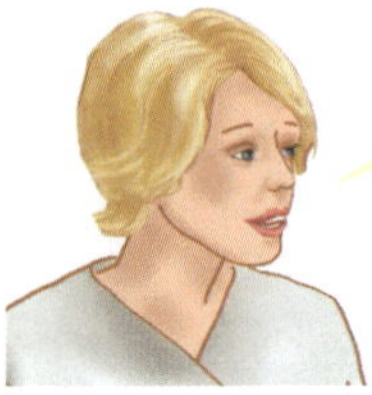

Patientin benötigt Erklärung des Formulars.

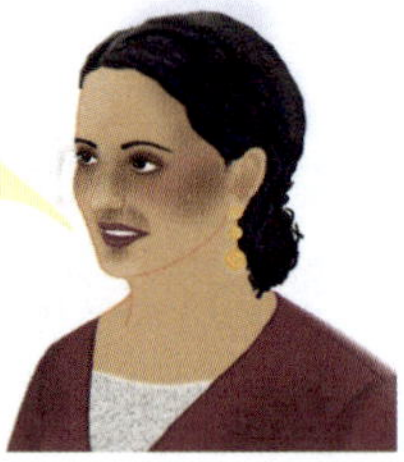

MFA erklärt, dass es sich um eine zeitliche Arbeitsunfähigkeitsbescheinigung handelt, die man bekommt, wenn man aus Krankheitsgründen nicht arbeitsfähig ist. Sie erklärt, welche Krankheitstage ausgewiesen sind.

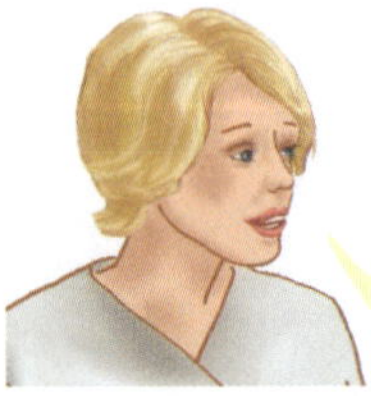

Patientin versteht nicht, warum sie es vor drei Monaten, als sie krank war, nicht bekam.

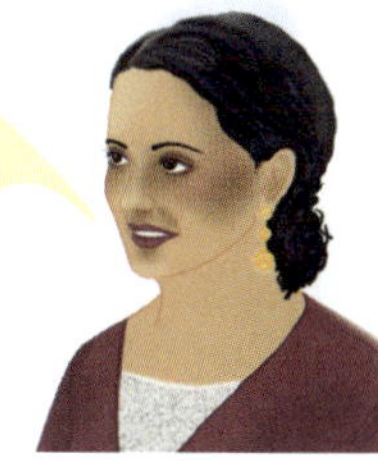

MFA fragt, wie lange sie damals krank war.

sick AE,
ill BE – krank

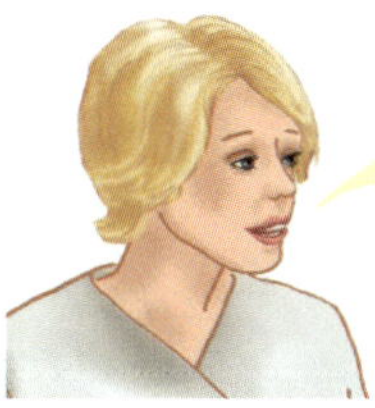

Patientin erinnert sich, dass es zwei Tage waren.

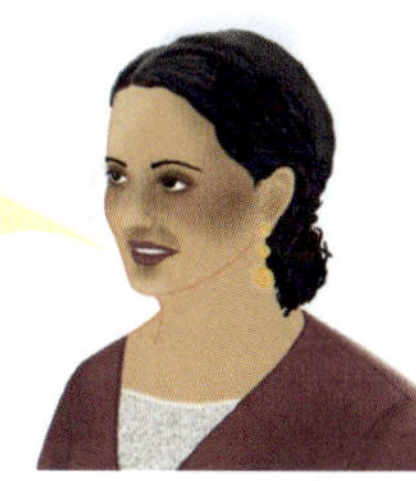

MFA erklärt, dass man eine AU normalerweise erst ab dem dritten Krankheitstag benötigt.

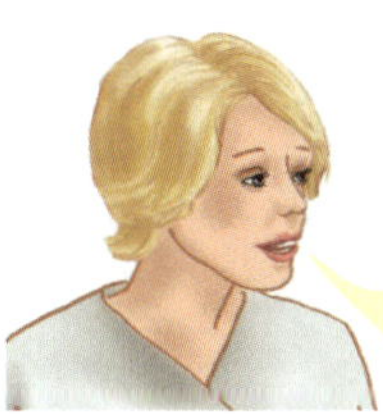

Patientin hat verstanden, fragt aber noch, was es mit den verschiedenen Formularen auf sich hat.

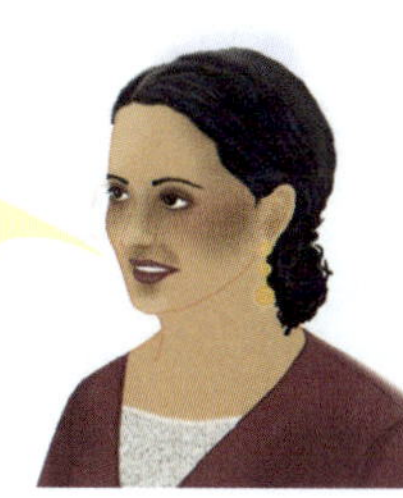

MFA klärt Patientin auf.

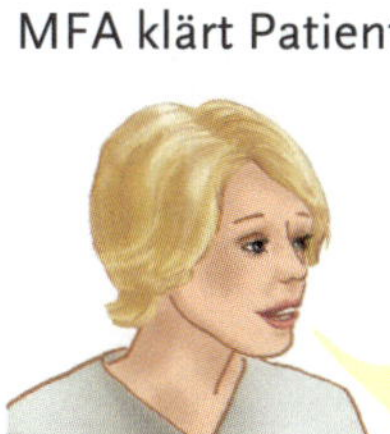

Patientin fragt erstaunt, ob ihr Chef dann nicht weiß, woran sie erkrankt ist.

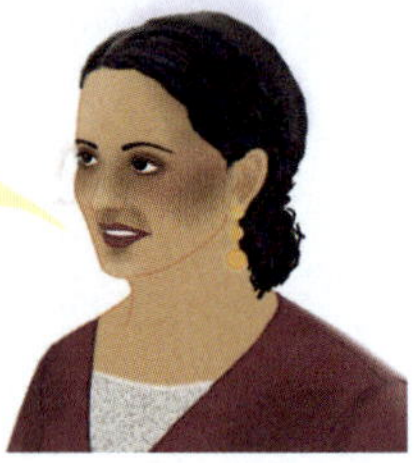

MFA bejaht.

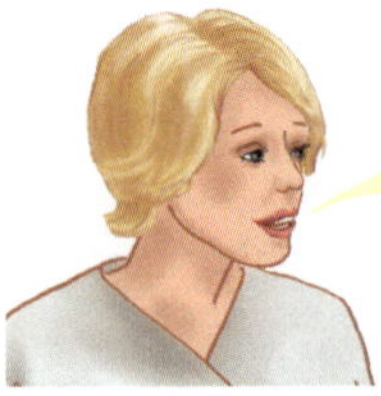

Patientin bedankt sich für die Auskunft und wünscht einen schönen Tag.

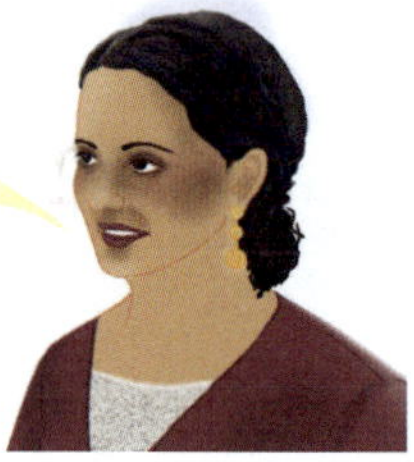

MFA antwortet und wünscht ebenfalls einen schönen Tag und gute Besserung.

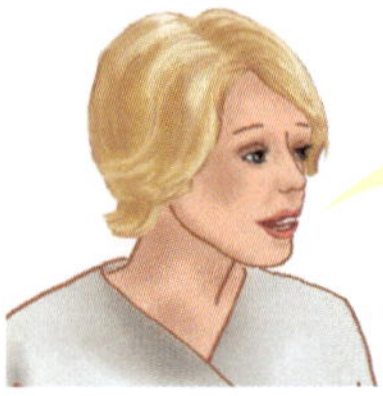

2 Preventive Health Check-ups

LISTENING Track 3

1 Listen to the dialog and answer the following questions:

- Why is the patient at the doctor's practice?
- What information does the medical assistant give?

READING

2 Read the following text and find the German words 3. Check any other new vocabulary in the vocabulary list or in a dictionary:

In Germany you can take advantage of routine preventive health check-ups. The costs are covered by health insurance. The same applies for standard immunizations.

Women and men aged over 35 can undergo health check-ups for circulatory, coronary, kidney and metabolic conditions every two years. This way, things like high blood pressure and diabetes can be detected and treated at an early stage.

Woman over 20 and men over 45 can undergo cancer check-ups every year. Many types of cancer can be fully cured if detected and treated at an early stage. The following cancer check-ups are recommended:

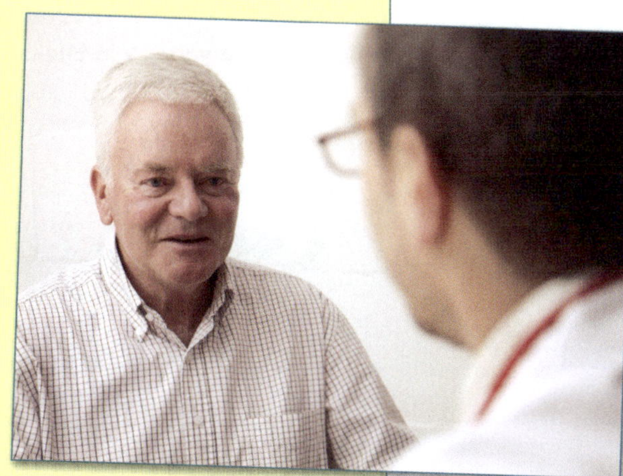

Women +20	Once a year: genital examination, smear test, irregularities in menstrual cycle
Women +30	Once a year: additional breast and skin examination, breast and lymph node screening, information for self-examination
Men +45	Once a year: prostate, genital and skin examination, palpation of the prostate gland and the lymph nodes
Women/Men +50	Once a year: large intestine and rectal examination to screen for potential cancer

Pregnant women should see a gynecologist regularly. They get a maternity record book in which all relevant data will be recorded.

After birth, the mother receives a personal child health record from the pediatrician in which all check-ups and standard vaccinations for the first 64 months of the baby's life (U1 – U9) are recorded.

Adults should undergo dental check-ups at least once a year, even if they do not have tooth pain. These routine dental check-ups are documented in a bonus booklet. If the patient needs a dental crown or bridge, the booklet has to be presented to the health insurance company.

immunization
circulatory
coronary
diabetes
irregularities
prostate
palpation
intestinal
examination
gynecologist
pediatrician
vaccination

COMPREHENSION

3 **Find the following words in the text:**

Vorteil nutzen — Vorsorgeuntersuchung — zutreffen auf

die Kosten tragen / decken — Impfung — sich unterziehen

Herz- — Kreislauf- — Stoffwechsel- — Nieren- — Zustand / Leiden

Bluthochdruck — feststellen — Frühstadium — Krebsvorsorge

heilen — Krone — Geburt — Brücke — Kinderarzt

Erwachsene — Kontrolluntersuchung der Zähne — mindestens

Beschwerden — Abstrich — Lymphknoten — Tastuntersuchung

Vorsteherdrüse — Dickdarmuntersuchung — Enddarmuntersuchung

4 **What would you say in English for these documents?**

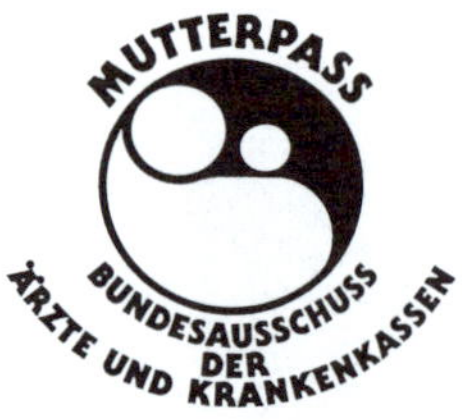

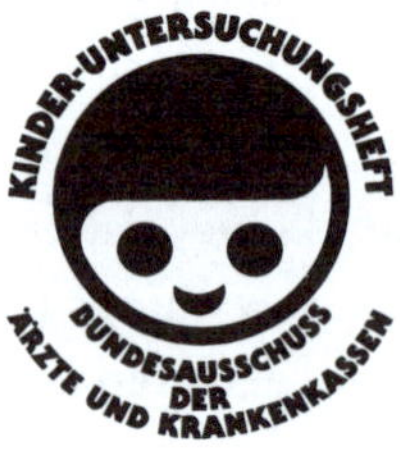

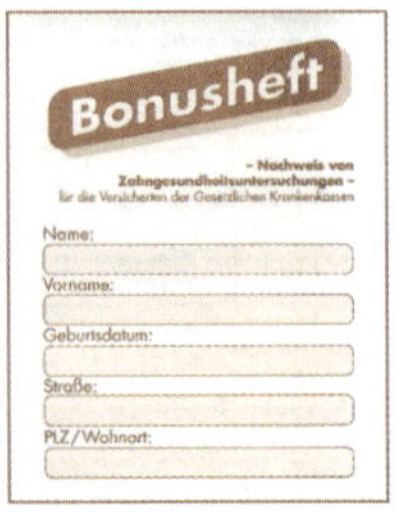

....

....

5 **True or false? Correct false statements:**

	T/F
1. The patient has to pay the costs for check-ups.	
2. The health insurance covers the costs for standard immunizations.	
3. When you are aged over 35 you can undergo check-ups for your heart, kidneys and metabolism.	
4. Breast screening is included in a routine cancer check-up for women over 20 years.	
5. A check-up of the prostate gland is recommended for women over 40.	
6. An examination of the large intestine and rectum is recommended from the age of 50.	
7. There is no particular document for pregnant women.	
8. Every newborn receives a bonus booklet for babies from the orthopedist.	
9. If you go to the dentist regularly every year the health insurance covers most of the costs for standard crowns and bridges.	

DIALOG / ROLEPLAY

6 **Write a dialog with a partner. Complete the speech bubbles:**

Jenny Mason wants to make an appointment for a cancer check-up for her 55 year old father:

Jenny möchte sich gerne über Krebsvorsorge für ihren 55-jährigen Vater informieren, da sie gehört hat, dass bei frühzeitiger Feststellung von Krebs die Heilungschancen besser sind.

....

....

....

....

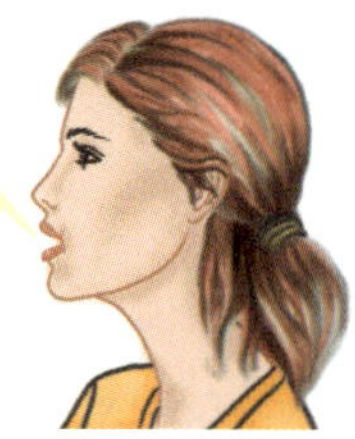

MFA bejaht und findet, dass die Menschen ab einem bestimmten Alter zur Krebsvorsorge gehen sollten. Sie bedauert, dass immer noch zu wenig Menschen das beachten.

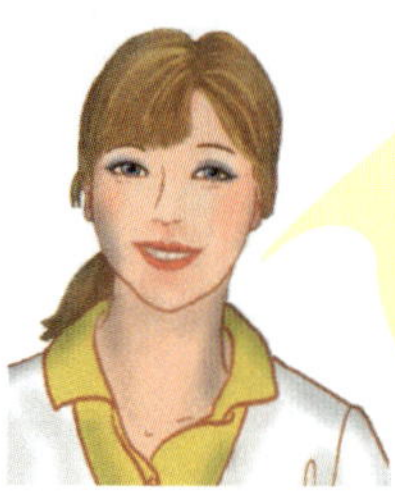

....

....

....

....

Jenny sagt, dass sie ihren Vater auch erst überzeugen (to convince) musste, bis er ihren Rat (advice) angenommen hat.

....

....

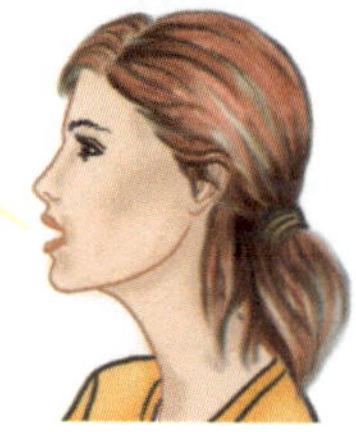

MFA fragt nach dem Alter des Vaters, da die Krebsvorsorgeuntersuchungen davon abhängen (to depend).

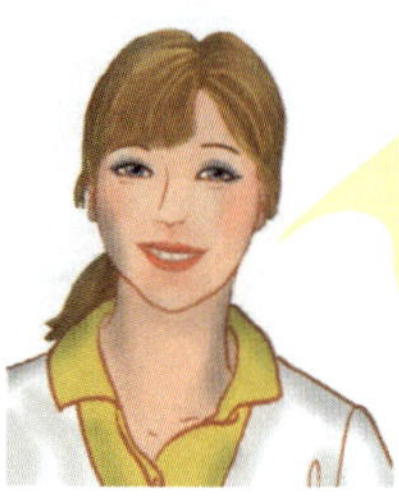

....

....

....

Jenny antwortet.

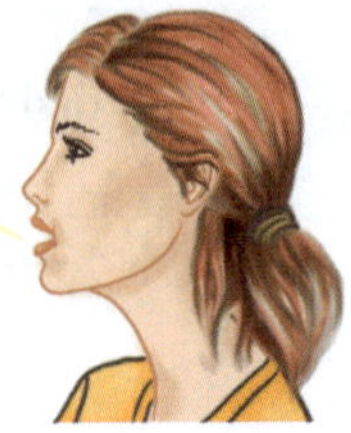

MFA fragt, ob irgendwelche Vorerkrankungen bestehen.

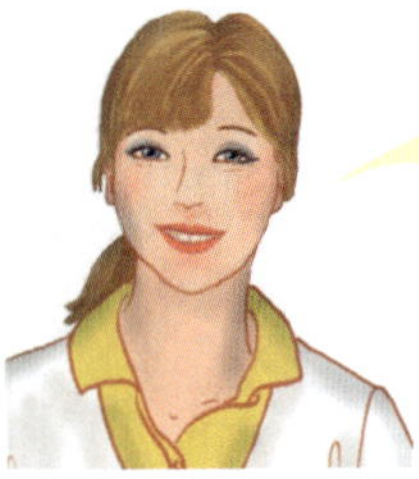

Jenny sagt, dass er an Diabetes leidet.

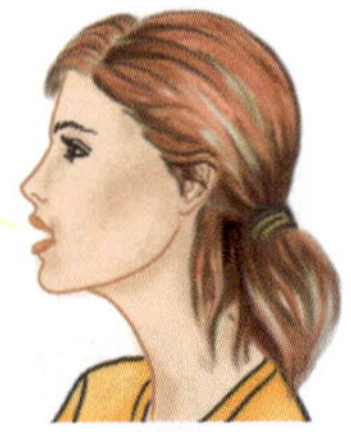

MFA nennt die möglichen Vorsorgeuntersuchungen für den Vater. Auch der Diabetes sollte beim Arzt genannt werden.

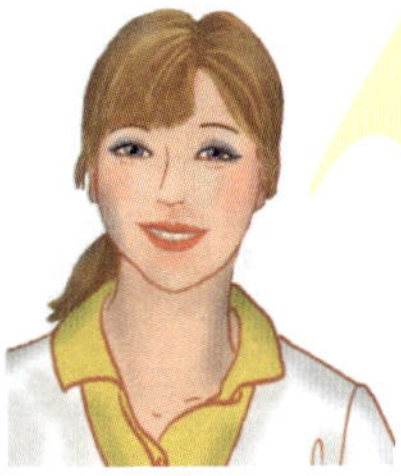

Jenny sagt, dass es sich nach einer umfangreichen (comprehensive) Untersuchung anhört. Sie bittet um einen Termin für ihren Vater.

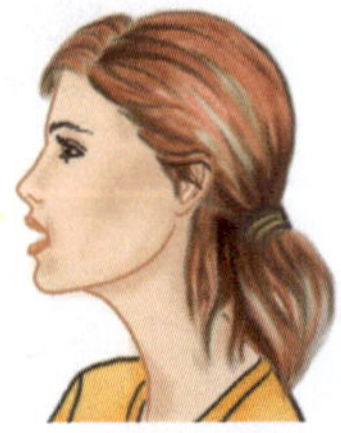

MFA bietet einen Termin genau in einer Woche um die selbe Zeit an.

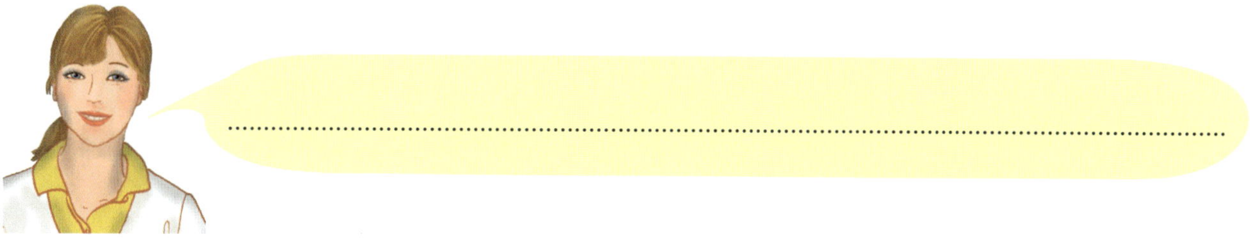

Jenny sagt, dass die Zeit ihm passen müsste.

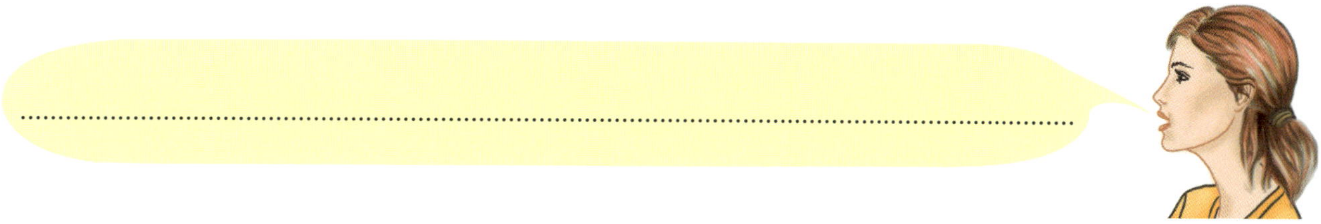

MFA benötigt seinen Namen und sagt, dass er seine Versichertenkarte mitbringen soll.
Sie übergibt die Notiz mit dem Termin.

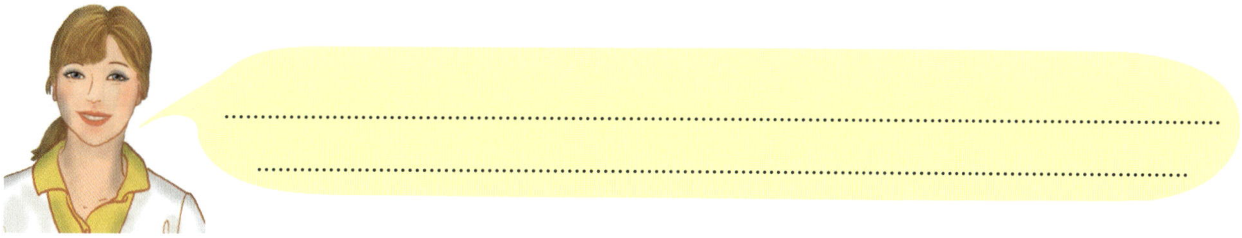

Jenny antwortet, bedankt sich für die Informationen und verabschiedet sich.

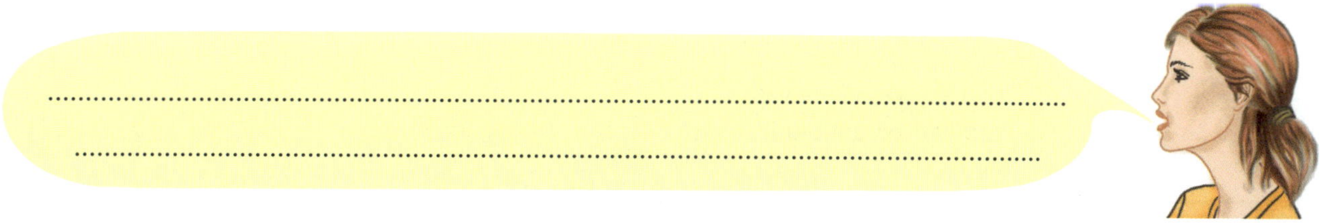

MFA antwortet und verabschiedet sich ebenfalls.

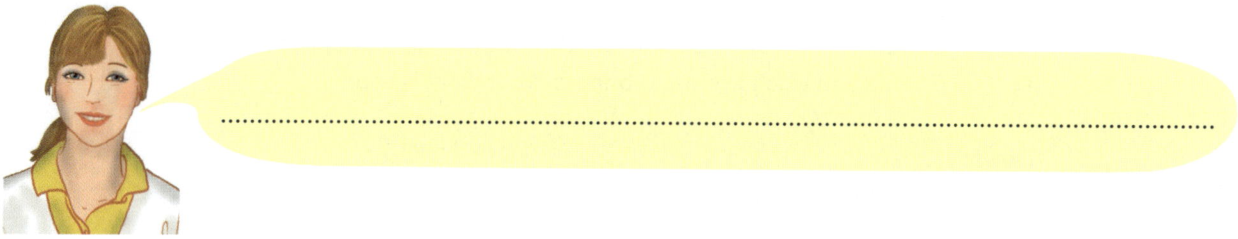

German Health Care System PUZZLE

7 **Fill in the crossword:**

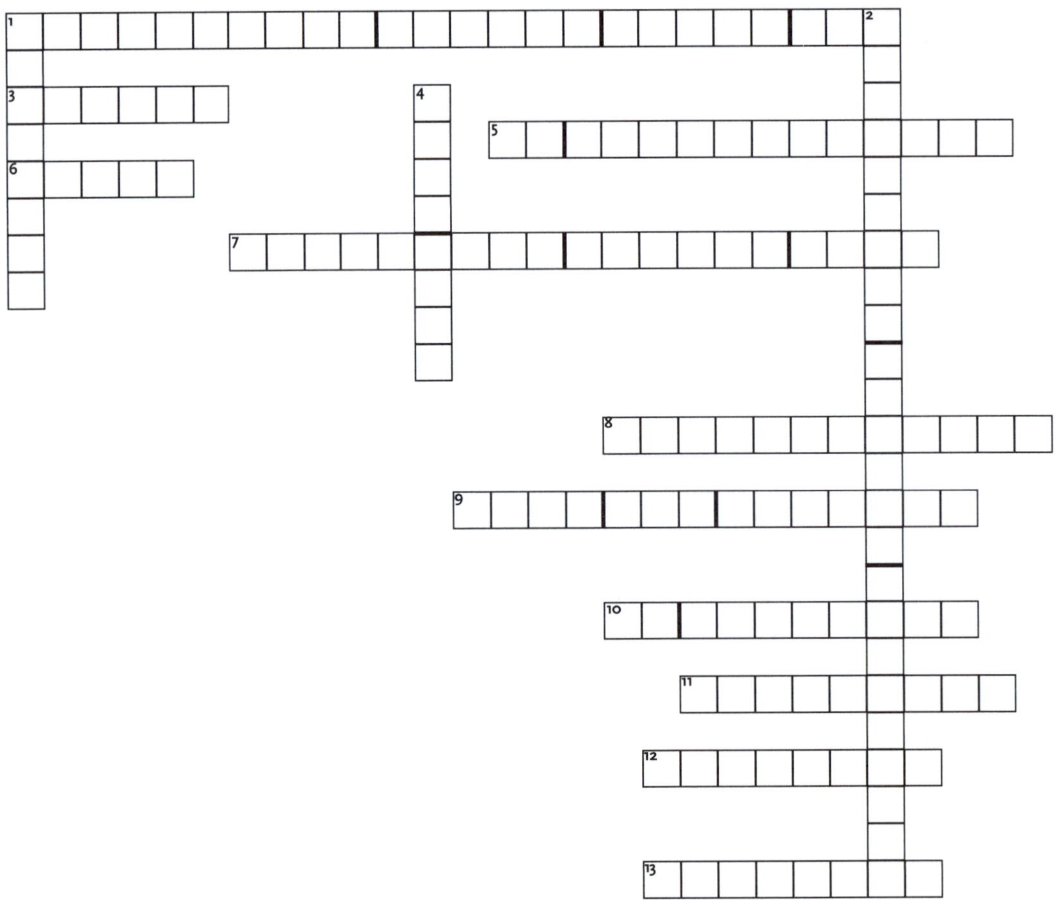

Across:

1 For early detection of diseases you should see the doctor for...
3 People over 18 are called...
5 You can get antibiotics only...
6 Person under 18 years
7 A pregnant woman gets this document
8 Another word for vaccination
9 Medicines you can buy without prescription are called... drugs
10 For medication on the pink prescription you have to make...
11 In 2. family members can be...
12 If a doctor thinks the patient should see another specialist he writes a...
13 The person who pays you money for your work is your...

Down:

1 You can buy medicines at the...
2 DAK, AOK are ...companies
4 If you are ill for more than three days you have to present a ... to your bos

3 Check-up 35+

LISTENING Track 4

1 Listen to the dialog and answer the following questions:

- *Why is Mrs. Pikker at the doctor's practice?*
- *What does the medical assistant do?*

READING

2 Read the following text and find the German words 3. Check any other new vocabulary in the vocabulary list or in a dictionary.

In Germany, from the age of 35 you may have a health check-up every two years in order to detect common illnesses like diabetes, cardiovascular or kidney disease early. There are a lot of risk factors for these diseases which should be avoided or at least reduced.

Your personal and your family's medical history are taken. The check-up includes a physical examination (including the head, neck, chest, abdomen, vertebral column and extremities). A blood and urine sample are taken to analyze your cholesterol and glucose levels and test your urine for protein, glucose, red and white blood cells. Your blood pressure is also taken.

The physician discusses the test results with you and gives you advice on how to change unhealthy habits. You do not have to pay the practice fee for this check-up.

If an illness is suspected or detected, the doctor will arrange further diagnostic tests or medical treatment.

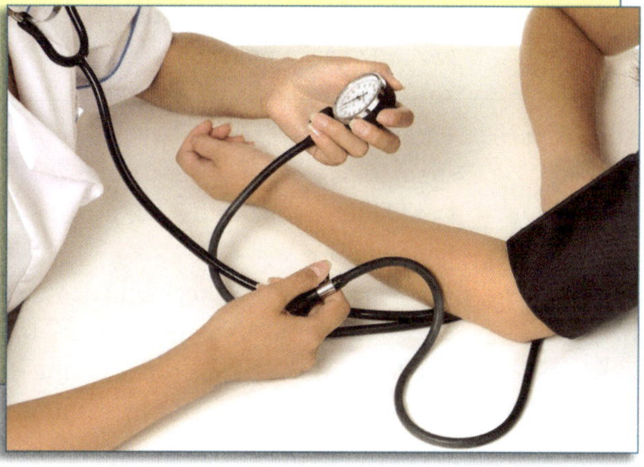

diabetes, cardiovascular, abdomen, vertebral column, urine, cholesterol, glucose, protein

physician AE, doctor BE und AE = Arzt

COMPREHENSION

3 Find the following words in the text:

Gesundheitsuntersuchung | auffinden | weitverbreitet/häufig vorkommend
Herz-Kreislauf-Erkrankung | Nierenerkrankung | Risikofaktoren
vermeiden | mindestens | Familienanamnese
körperliche Untersuchung | Wirbelsäule | Bauch | Brustkorb
Blutprobe | Urinprobe | Blut-Cholesterin-Spiegel | Eiweiß
Blutglukosespiegel | Blutdruck | messen | Arzt
Untersuchungsergebnisse | Rat | ungesunde Gewohnheiten

4 **Answer the following questions:**

1. From what age does the health insurance pay for this check-up?
2. What are the reasons for this check-up?
3. What does the check-up include and what does the medical assistant / doctor do?

READING Track 4

5 **Now read the dialog again and check the German words 6. Check any other new vocabulary in the vocabulary list or in a dictionary.**

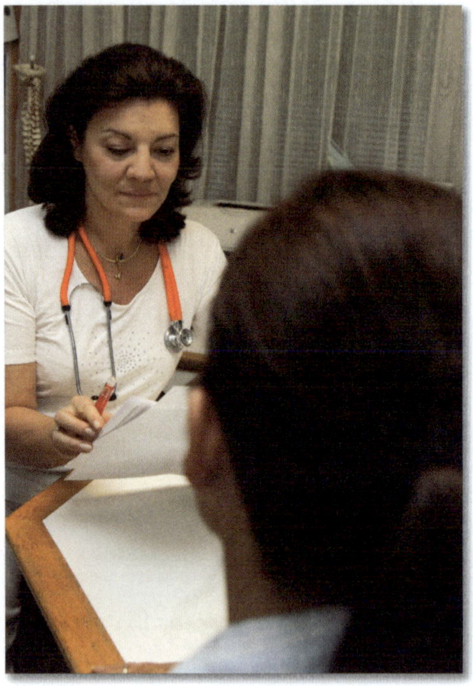

MA: Guten Morgen. Was kann ich für Sie tun?

PATIENT: Sorry, my German is still pretty bad. Do you speak English?

MA: Yes, how can I help you?

PATIENT: I am Elena Pikker and I have an appointment for a general check-up at 8:30.

MA: Could I have your chip card, please?

PATIENT: Here you are.

MA: Mrs. Pikker, for the check-up I need a midstream urine sample. Here is a urine cup for you. The bathroom is on the right hand side next to the entrance. Put the urine sample in the little window. Do you know how to collect it?

PATIENT: Yes, I've often had to do it because of my bladder inflammations.

MA: Could you then take a seat in the laboratory just over there, please? I'll be with you in a minute.

(...)

PATIENT: Ok.

MA: So Mrs. Pikker, first of all I'm going to take your blood pressure. Could you take off your jacket and pullover, please? You can put your clothes on the empty chair.

PATIENT: Yes, of course.

MA: Now, I'm going to wrap the cuff around your arm and pump it up. It might feel a little bit tight for a moment... 150 over 100.

PATIENT: Is my blood pressure OK?

MA: It's a bit high. But the doctor will discuss it with you. Do you or anyone in your family suffer from high blood pressure?

PATIENT: My blood pressure has always been normal as far as I remember. But my grandparents on my mother's side had hypertension.

MA: I see. Now, I have to take some blood to check your cholesterol and glucose levels. First I need to find a good vein. I 'm now going to fasten the tourniquet. Could you clench a fist, please? Oh, here is a good one. I need to disinfect the injection site, it'll feel a bit cold. Are you alright Mrs. Pikker?

PATIENT: Yes, I'm fine.

MA: So, now the needle, it might hurt a little... So, I'm done. Please press the swab on the injection site for a while. Do you bruise easily Mrs. Pikker?

PATIENT: Yes, I do.

MA: Then I'll put a little pressure on it with a band-aid. That's it. Leave it on for at least an hour. Before you see the doctor I need to ask you some questions. Do you or anyone in your family have coronary heart disease or peripheral arterial disease?

PATIENT: No, I don't. I don't know about my family.

MA: Do you or anyone in your family suffer from diabetes?

PATIENT: I don't have diabetes, but my grandfather has had an increased blood glucose level for some years now.

MA: And what about high blood fats?

PATIENT: I think he also has high cholesterol. But I don't know about my blood fats.

MA: Well, we'll find out with your blood sample. Is there a history of kidney disease in your family?

PATIENT: No, I don't think so.

MA: And what about lung disease?

PATIENT: My father has asthma. I cough a bit now and then.

MA: Do you smoke Mrs. Pikker?

PATIENT: Yes, I do.

MA: How many cigarettes a day?

PATIENT: About a pack. I know I should quit. But so much stress, you know...

MA: I see. So would you say it is constant emotional stress?

PATIENT: You know, my life is not easy. I'm a single mother and have to work a lot to support me and my family...

MA: Oh dear. Life is not always easy, is it? And what about alcohol Mrs. Pikker?

PATIENT: Oh, I don't drink a lot. One or two glasses of wine a week.

MA: One last question: Do you exercise regularly?

PATIENT: No, I just don't have the time.

MA: Ok Mrs. Pikker, the doctor still has to examine you. Please take a seat in the waiting-room. He'll call you.

PATIENT: When will the blood test results be in?

MA: In two days. We are going to make another appointment so that you can discuss the results with the doctor.

COMPREHENSION

6 **Find the following words in the text:**

Mittelstrahlurin | Urinbecher | Blasenentzündung

Blutdruckmanschette | eng | besprechen | Bluthochdruck

Vene | Stauschlauch | eine Faust machen | desinfizieren

Injektionsstelle/Einstichstelle | schmerzen/weh tun | Tupfer

Blutergüsse bekommen | Pflaster | Blutfette | koronare Herzkrankheit

husten | Sport treiben | alleinerziehende Mutter

7 Fill in the German form ("Berichtsvordruck Gesundheitsuntersuchung") with the information you now have:

Berichtsvordruck Gesundheitsuntersuchung

Teil a (mit der Abrechnung der KV zuleiten)

Beleg nicht knicken!

Beleg-Nr. 27377134

Krankenkasse

AOK [X] BKK [ ] IKK [ ]
Landwirtsch. Krankenkasse [ ] Bundes-knappschaft [ ]
VdAK [ ] AEV [ ]

Alter

unter 35 [ ] 50–54 [ ] 70–74 [ ]
35–39 [ ] 55–59 [ ] 75–79 [ ]
40–44 [ ] 60–64 [ ] 80 u. älter [ ]
45–49 [ ] 65–69 [ ]

Geschlecht weiblich [ ] männlich [ ]

Es wird gleichzeitig eine Krebsfrüherkennungs-untersuchung durchgeführt? ja [ ]

Anamnese

Es wurde bereits eine Gesundheitsuntersuchung nach den Richtlinien durchgeführt? ja [ ]

Vorbestehende Krankheiten

	in der Eigen-anamnese	in der Familien-anamnese
Hypertonie	[ ]	[ ]
koronare Herzkrankheit	[ ]	[ ]
sonst. arter. Verschlußkrankheit	[ ]	[ ]
Diabetes mellitus	[ ]	[ ]
Hyperlipidämie	[ ]	[ ]
Nierenkrankheiten	[ ]	[ ]
Lungenerkrankung	[ ]	[ ]

Persönliche Risikofaktoren

Nikotinabusus [ ] Adipositas [ ]
dauerhafte emotionale Belastungsfaktoren [ ] Alkoholabusus [ ]
Bewegungsmangel [ ]

Arztstempel

Befunde

krankhafte Veränderungen (ohne interkurrente Befunde)

Brustkorb (Inspektion) [ ] Bewegungs-apparat [ ]
Herzauskultation [ ] Haut [ ]
Lungenauskultation [ ] Sinnesorgane [ ]
Abdomenpalpation (einschl. Nierenlager) [ ] Nervensystem [ ]
Fußpulse [ ] Psyche [ ]
Karotisauskultation [ ]

Blutdruck

bis 140/90 mmHg [ ] bis 180/105 mmHg [ ]
bis 160/95 mmHg [ ] über 180/105 mmHg [ ]

Der relativ höhere Wert (systolisch oder diastolisch) bestimmt die Klassenzugehörigkeit (z.B.: 150/100 mmHg= bis 180/105 mmHg). Bei Werten über 140/90 mmHg ist eine zweite Messung durchzuführen und der Mittelwert aus beiden Messungen für die Klassenzuordnung zugrunde zu legen.

Labor

Blut

Gesamtcholesterin:
bis 200 mg/dl [ ]
201 bis 220 mg/dl [ ]
221 bis 250 mg/dl [ ]
251 bis 300 mg/dl [ ]
über 300 mg/dl [ ]

Bestimmung des HDL/LDL-Cholesterins veranlaßt? ja [ ]

Glukosewert auffällig? ja [ ]

Harn

Eiweiß positiv [ ] Ery/Hb positiv [ ] Leukozyten positiv [ ]
Glukose positiv [ ] Nitrit positiv [ ]

Neue Diagnose / Verdachtsdiagnose

(ohne interkurrente Erkrankungen)

	neu gestellte Diagnose	davon behandlungs-bedürftig	Abklärungs-diagnostik bei Verdacht auf bisher unbekannte Erkrankung eingeleitet
Hypertonie	[ ]	[ ]	[ ]
koronare Herzkrankheit	[ ]	[ ]	[ ]
arterielle Verschlußkrankheit	[ ]	[ ]	[ ]
Diabetes mellitus	[ ]	[ ]	[ ]
Hyperlipidämie	[ ]	[ ]	[ ]
Nieren-erkrankung	[ ]	[ ]	[ ]
Lungen-erkrankung	[ ]	[ ]	[ ]
orthopädische Erkrankung	[ ]	[ ]	[ ]
Haut-erkrankung	[ ]	[ ]	[ ]
Erkrankung des Nervensystems	[ ]	[ ]	[ ]
Erkrankung der Psyche	[ ]	[ ]	[ ]
andere Krankheiten	[ ]	[ ]	[ ]

Folgende Maßnahmen wurden veranlaßt

Ernährungs-umstellg./Diätber. [ ] neu verordnete medikamentöse Therapie [ ]
Nikotin-entwöhnung [ ] sonstiges [ ]
Bewegungs-training [ ] keine speziellen Maßnahmen [ ]
Entspannungs-techniken [ ]

Dieser Beleg kann manuell oder maschinell ausgefüllt werden.
Den Beleg nur mit schwarzem oder blauem Kugelschreiber ausfüllen.

[X] Bitte so ausfüllen

Name: Elena Pikker

Geburtsdatum: 12.08.1974

8 **Correct these false statements:**

1. Mrs. Pikker has an appointment at half past nine.

....

2. The medical assistant needs a stool sample from the patient.

....

3. The medical assistant asks the patient to take off her trousers to take the blood pressure.

....

....

4. A tourniquet is used to measure the blood pressure.

....

5. Mrs. Pikker's blood pressure is 100/70 which is too low.

....

6. Mrs. Pikker has a family history of hypotension.

....

7. The medical assistant first disinfects the injection site, then looks for a good vein, then inserts the needle, then fastens the cuff and then puts a band-aid on the injection site.

....

....

....

8. Taking blood does not hurt at all.

....

9. Mrs. Pikker has bruises on her arm.

....

10. Mrs. Pikker has no family history of diabetes, high blood fats, kidney and lung disease.

....

....

Berichtsvordruck Gesundheitsuntersuchung

Teil a (mit der Abrechnung der KV zuleiten)

Beleg nicht knicken!

Beleg-Nr. 27377134

Krankenkasse

AOK [X] BKK [ ] IKK [ ]

Landwirtsch. Krankenkasse [ ] Bundes-knappschaft [ ]

VdAK [ ] AEV [ ]

Alter

unter 35 [ ] 50–54 [X] 70–74 [ ]

35–39 [ ] 55–59 [ ] 75–79 [ ]

40–44 [ ] 60–64 [ ] 80 u. älter [ ]

45–49 [ ] 65–69 [ ]

Geschlecht

weiblich [ ] männlich [X]

Es wird gleichzeitig eine Krebsfrüherkennungs-untersuchung durchgeführt? ja [ ]

Anamnese

Es wurde bereits eine Gesundheitsuntersuchung nach den Richtlinien durchgeführt? ja [ ]

Vorbestehende Krankheiten

	in der Eigen-anamnese	in der Familien-anamnese
Hypertonie	[ ]	[X]
koronare Herzkrankheit	[ ]	[ ]
sonst. arter. Verschlußkrankheit	[ ]	[ ]
Diabetes mellitus	[ ]	[X]
Hyperlipidämie	[ ]	[X]
Nierenkrankheiten	[ ]	[ ]
Lungenerkrankung	[ ]	[ ]

Persönliche Risikofaktoren

Nikotinabusus [ ] Adipositas [ ]

dauerhafte emotionale Belastungsfaktoren [X] Alkoholabusus [ ]

Bewegungsmangel [ ]

Arztstempel

Befunde

krankhafte Veränderungen (ohne interkurrente Befunde)

Brustkorb (Inspektion) [ ] Bewegungs-apparat [ ]

Herzauskultation [ ] Haut [ ]

Lungenauskultation [ ] Sinnesorgane [ ]

Abdomenpalpation (einschl. Nierenlager) [ ] Nervensystem [ ]

Fußpulse [ ] Psyche [ ]

Karotisauskultation [ ]

Blutdruck

bis 140/90 mmHg [ ] bis 180/105 mmHg [X]

bis 160/95 mmHg [ ] über 180/105 mmHg [ ]

Der relativ höhere Wert (systolisch oder diastolisch) bestimmt die Klassenzugehörigkeit (z.B.: 150/100 mmHg= bis 180/105 mmHg). Bei Werten über 140/90 mmHg ist eine zweite Messung durchzuführen und der Mittelwert aus beiden Messungen für die Klassenzuordnung zugrunde zu legen.

Labor

Blut

Gesamtcholesterin:

bis 200 mg/dl [ ]

201 bis 220 mg/dl [ ]

221 bis 250 mg/dl [ ]

251 bis 300 mg/dl [ ]

über 300 mg/dl [ ]

Bestimmung des HDL/LDL-Cholesterins veranlaßt? ja [ ]

Glukosewert auffällig? ja [ ]

Harn

Eiweiß positiv [ ] Ery/Hb positiv [ ] Leukozyten positiv [ ]

Glukose positiv [ ] Nitrit positiv [ ]

Dieser Beleg kann manuell oder maschinell ausgefüllt werden.
Den Beleg nur mit schwarzem oder blauem Kugelschreiber ausfüllen.

[X] Bitte so ausfüllen

Neue Diagnose / Verdachtsdiagnose

(ohne interkurrente Erkrankungen)

	neu gestellte Diagnose	davon behandlungs-bedürftig	Abklärungs-diagnostik bei Verdacht auf bisher unbekannte Erkrankung eingeleitet
Hypertonie	[ ]	[ ]	[ ]
koronare Herzkrankheit	[ ]	[ ]	[ ]
arterielle Ver-schlußkrankheit	[ ]	[ ]	[ ]
Diabetes mellitus	[ ]	[ ]	[ ]
Hyperlipidämie	[ ]	[ ]	[ ]
Nieren-erkrankung	[ ]	[ ]	[ ]
Lungen-erkrankung	[ ]	[ ]	[ ]
orthopädische Erkrankung	[ ]	[ ]	[ ]
Haut-erkrankung	[ ]	[ ]	[ ]
Erkrankung des Nervensystems	[ ]	[ ]	[ ]
Erkrankung der Psyche	[ ]	[ ]	[ ]
andere Krankheiten	[ ]	[ ]	[ ]

Folgende Maßnahmen wurden veranlaßt

Ernährungs-umstellg./Diätber. [ ] neu verordnete medikamentöse Therapie [ ]

Nikotin-entwöhnung [ ] sonstiges [ ]

Bewegungs-training [ ] keine speziellen Maßnahmen [ ]

Entspannungs-techniken [ ]

Name: Benjamin Black

Geburtsdatum: 30.11.1959

DIALOG

9 **Above is Benjamin Black's form which has been filled in by a medical assistant. Write a dialog.**

At the reception

MFA begrüßt den Patienten.

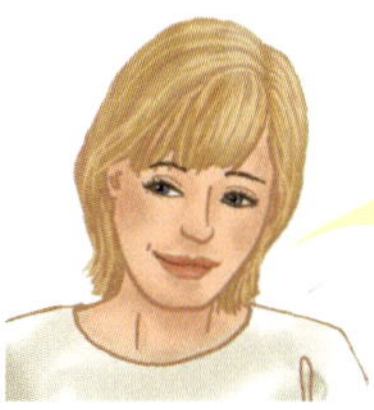

Der Patient stellt sich vor. Er hat einen Termin um 8:15 Uhr zur Gesundheitsuntersuchung.

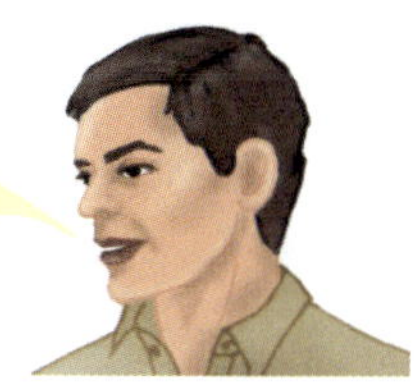

MFA bittet um die KVK, sie bittet den Patienten um Gewinnung einer Urinprobe und erklärt, wo er diese hinstellen soll. Er soll anschließend vor dem Labor warten.

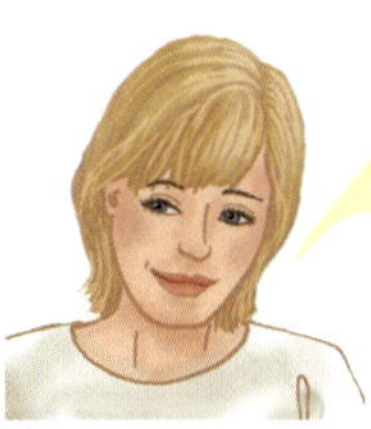

MFA gibt ihm seine Karte wieder.

At the laboratory / Measuring blood pressure

MFA bittet den Patienten, im Labor Platz zu nehmen. Sie möchte zunächst seinen Blutdruck messen und fragt ihn, ob er oder jemand in der Familie an Bluthochdruck leidet.

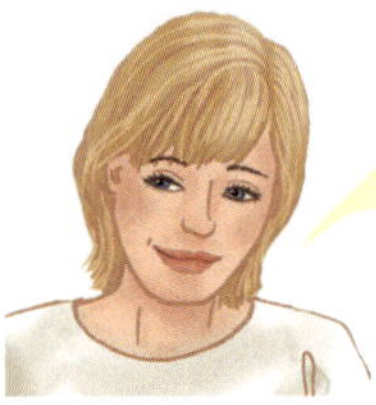

Der Patient antwortet (siehe Vordruck Benjamin Black).

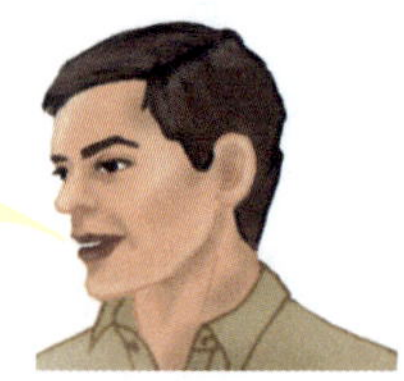

MFA gibt entsprechende Anweisungen und erklärt dem Patienten, was sie tut...
Sie teilt ihm den Wert mit.

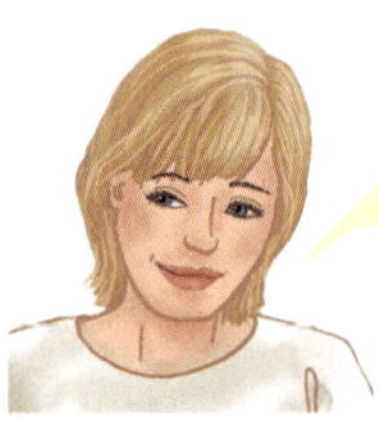

Der Patient fragt, ob der Wert o.k. ist.

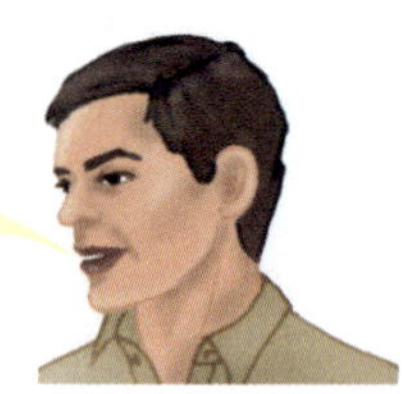

MFA antwortet.

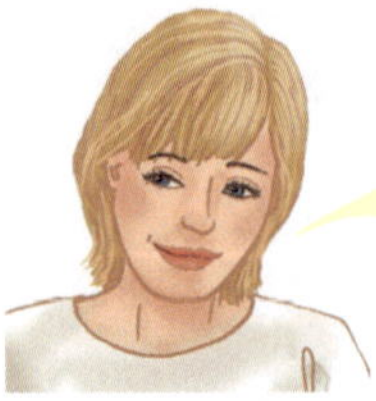

Taking blood

MFA teilt mit, dass sie ihm zur Bestimmung des Blutzuckers und der Blutfette Blut abnehmen muss. Sie fragt nach der Krankenvorgeschichte bezüglich Diabetes und hoher Cholesterinwerte.

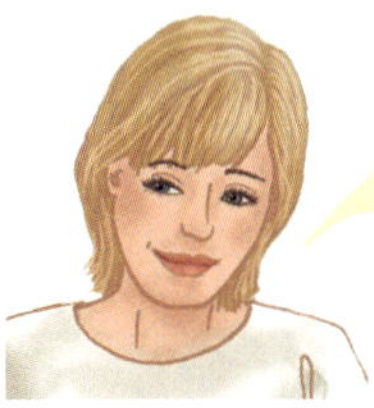

Der Patient antwortet (siehe Vordruck). Er sagt, dass ihm bei der BE meist schwindelig wird.

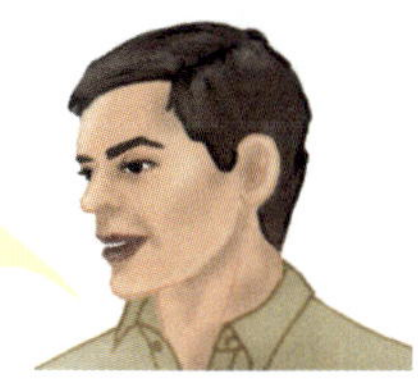

MFA reagiert entsprechend. Dann kommentiert sie die Blutentnahme. Zwischendurch erkundigt sie sich nach dem Befinden des Patienten.

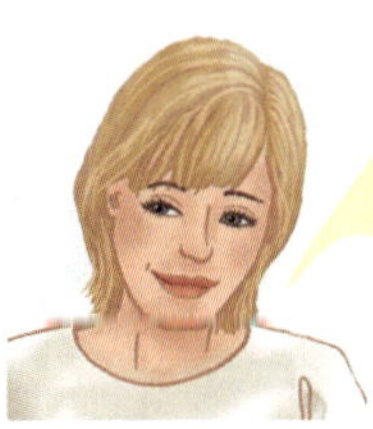

Der Patient antwortet.

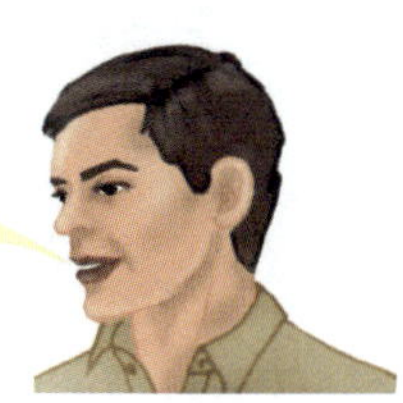

Taking a medical history

MFA ist fertig, lobt den Patienten und teilt ihm mit, dass sie ihm noch einige Fragen bezüglich seiner Krankenvorgeschichte und persönlicher Risikofaktoren stellen muss. Zunächst fragt sie nach KHK.

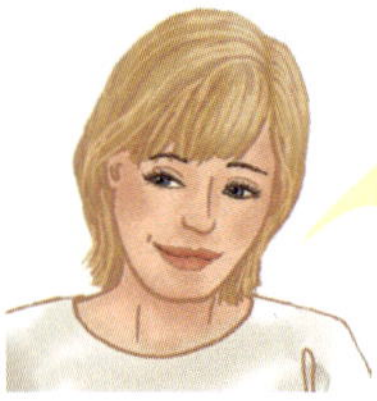

Der Patient antwortet (siehe Vordruck).

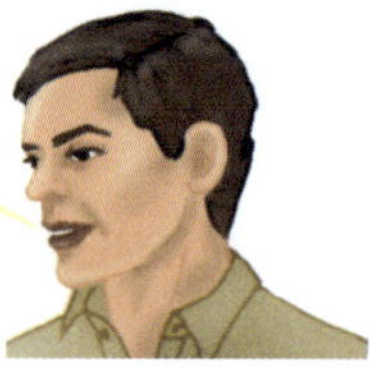

MFA fragt nach Nieren- und Lungenerkrankungen.

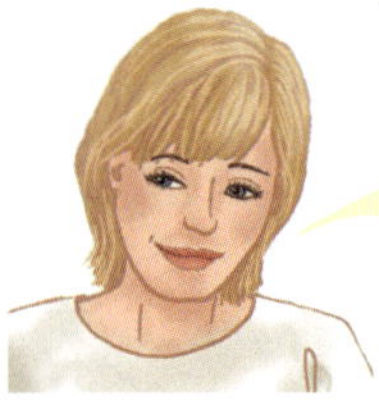

Der Patient antwortet (siehe Vordruck).

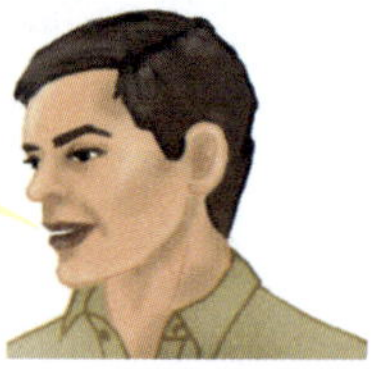

MFA fragt nach Rauchverhalten.

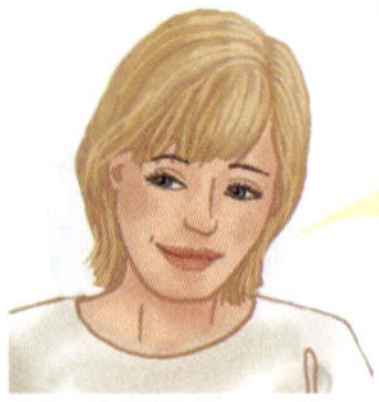

Der Patient antwortet (siehe Vordruck).

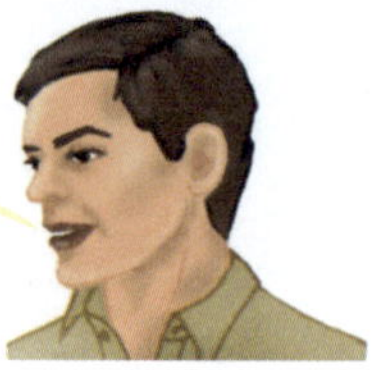

MFA fragt nach Alkohol.

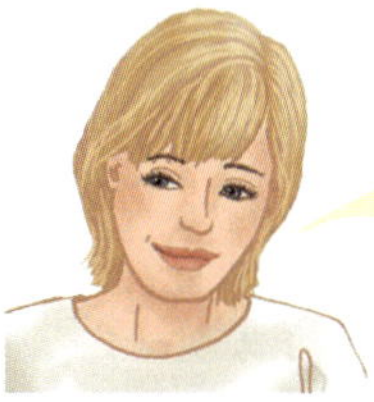

Der Patient antwortet (siehe Vordruck).

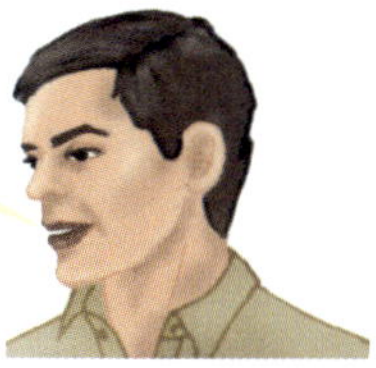

MFA fragt nach Stressfaktoren.

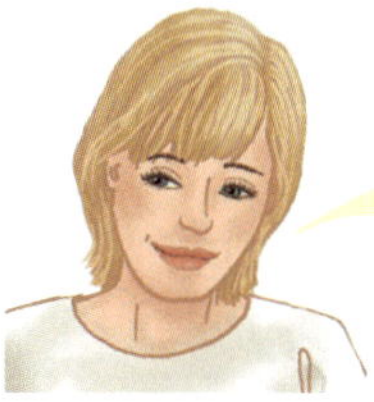

Der Patient nennt einen Faktor, der ihn zur Zeit sehr belastet.

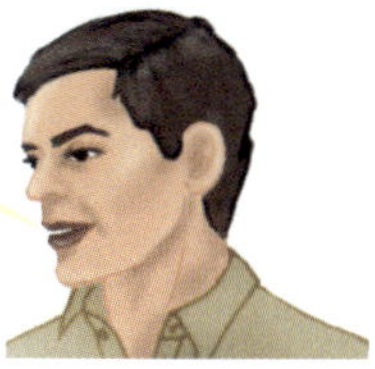

MFA fragt, ob er regelmäßig Sport treibt.

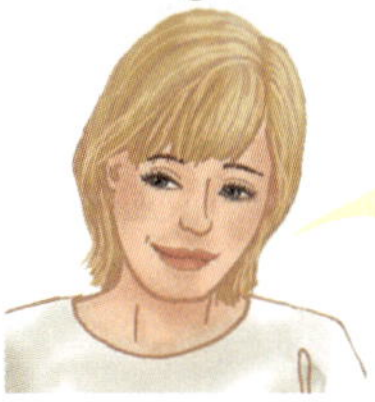

Der Patient geht zweimal die Woche ins Fitnessstudio und Joggen.

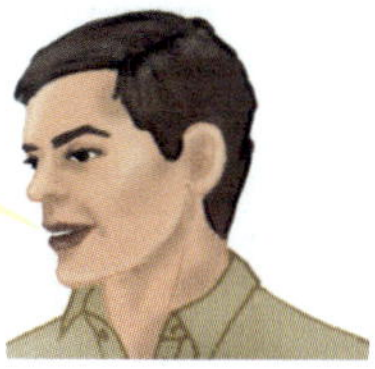

MFA teilt dem Patienten mit, dass der Arzt ihn gleich untersuchen wird und er noch kurz im Wartezimmer Platz nehmen soll.

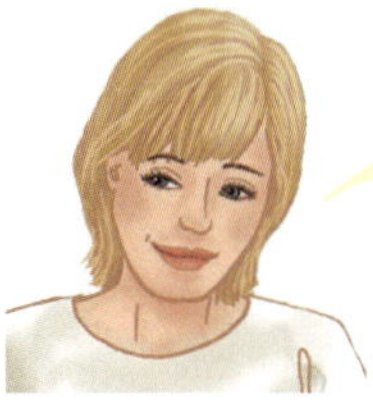

HEALTH CHECK-UP WORD SEARCH

10 **Can you find 33 hidden words? Find the hidden message in the remaining letters:**

H Y A V O I D T R S I S K T F E A C
A I R T O R C S T W S S T O Z R C Z
B K G O Y E V E R A Y S E U D U Q L
I I U H T Y H H U B I T V R I S D O
T D C E B S R C H F I F B N S A I R
W N D B V L I A A S C L J I I E S E
E E C N R F O H N T O U N Q N M C T
S Y W N M U C O L O R F P U F O U S
I N I E V N I N D A R A J E E K S E
C C B A E T P S A P C O E T C Q S L
R O G L C U A J E I R I C H T M M O
E F C E Z M A D V I C E D J S G E H
X E J N P H E A R T D I S E A S E C
E N T L U S E R T S E T S S M E E F
I L E V E L E S O C U L G Y U U X F
U R I N E S A M P L E S D V H R O U
Y H T L A E H N U C H E C K U P E C
D I A B E T E S T D O A B D O M E N

Hidden message: ....

4 Treatment of a Sprained Ankle

LISTENING Track 5

1 **Listen to the dialog and answer the following questions:**

- *Why is the patient at the doctor's practice?*
- *What is the medical assistant doing?*

READING

2 **Read the following text and find the German words 3. Check any other new vocabulary in the vocabulary list or in a dictionary.**

A **sprain** is an **injury** to **ligaments** surrounding a **joint**. Ligaments attach[1] bones to each other and give support[2] to joints. Sprains are usually the result of **twisting** the joint and are sometimes so severe[3] that a **fracture** may also occur[4]. This can be diagnosed by taking an X-ray image (radiography). Sprains most commonly occur to the **ankle**. The joint may be swollen and bruised. The patient has pain and difficulties walking. Following a sprain, the **advice** is "to pay the PRICE" (Protection, Rest, Ice, Compression, Elevation[5]) and avoid "HARM" (Heat, Alcohol, Running, Massage) for the first three days. An **elastic bandage** or **crutches** for ankle sprains can give support. **Painkillers** and physiotherapy may also be needed. **Surgery** is sometimes needed if a ligament ruptures[6]. The aim of the treatment is to reduce **inflammation**, **swelling** and pain to a minimum.

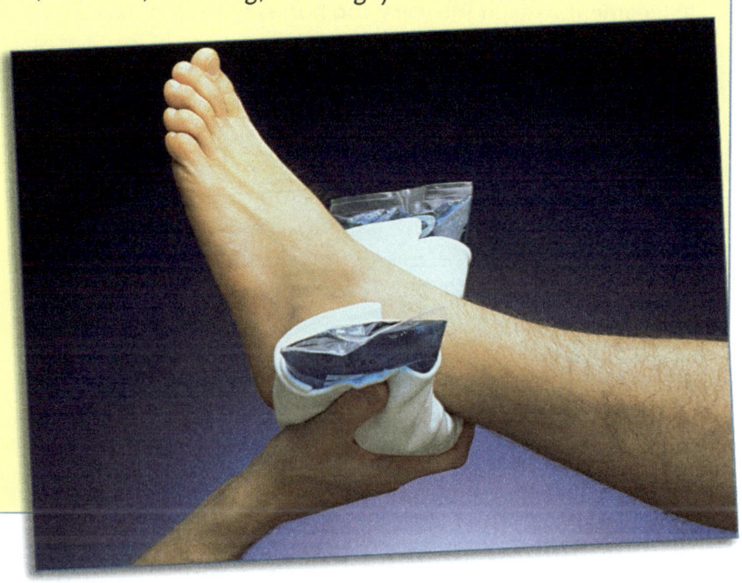

ligaments, radiography, massage, crutches, physiotherapy, surgery

1 to attach – befestigen
2 support – Halt, Unterstützung
3 severe – schwerwiegend
4 to occur – auftreten, vorkommen
5 elevation – hier: Hochlagerung
6 to rupture – reißen

Do's

P – Protect the injured part from further injury.
R – Rest the affected joint for 48 – 72 hours.
I – an ice pack should be put on the injury every two hours for 10-30 minutes a time to limit pain and inflammation.
C – Compression with a bandage limits swelling and helps to rest the joint.
E – Elevate the sprained body part to reduce swelling, that means that when you have a sprained ankle you should keep the foot up.

Don'ts

H – Heat increases the blood flow and inflammation in the first three days.
A – Alcohol increases bleeding and swelling.
R – Running and exercising can cause more damage.
M – Massage increases bleeding and swelling in the first three days.

COMPREHENSION

3 **Find the following words in the text:**

Gelenk · Knochenbruch · Unterarmgehhilfe · Verletzung · Operation · Verstauchung · Entzündung · Bänder · Schwellung · Schaden · begrenzen · Blutfluss · hoch lagern · Blutung · verstärken/erhöhen · Krankengymnastik · Verband · Ruhe · Schmerzmittel · Druck · Knöchel

4 **Are the following statements true or false? Correct false statements:**

	T/F
1. An injury of ligaments is called a sprain.	
2. Ligaments attach muscles and bones to each other.	
3. Most sprains happen to the wrist.	
4. You should apply heat to treat a sprained ankle in the beginning.	
5. Crutches and elastic bandages help to rest the ankle.	
6. Swelling can be reduced by compression and running.	
7. Swelling can be reduced by keeping the foot up.	
8. The patient should drink a little alcohol to kill the pain.	

DIALOG / ROLEPLAY

5 **Write a dialog with a partner. Fill in the speech bubbles:**

Yesterday Mr. Amin twisted his left ankle when he walked downstairs. He didn't go to see the doctor because he thought it wasn't too bad. However, today his ankle is swollen, bruised and he can hardly walk because it just hurts so much. He called his friend who drove him to the orthopedist.

At the reception

MFA begrüßt den Patienten und fragt, was sie für ihn tun kann.

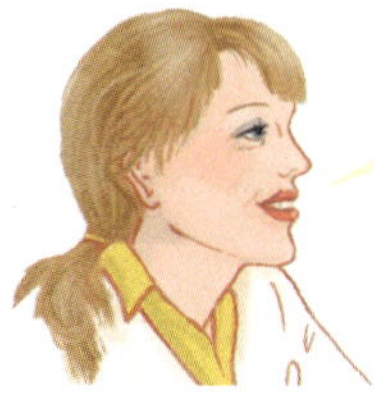

Patient stellt sich vor und beschreibt, was passiert ist.

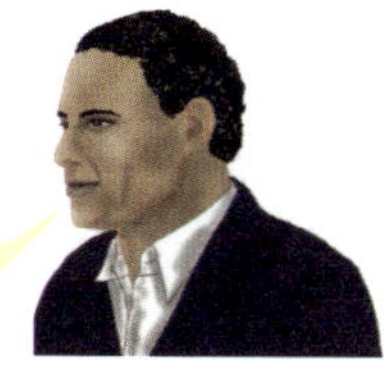

MFA stützt Patient und hilft ihm ins Wartezimmer. Sie bemerkt, dass der Fuß sehr dick und blau ist. Nachdem er sitzt und den Fuß hochgelagert hat, fragt die MFA nach der Versichertenkarte und 10,- Euro Praxisgebühr. Sie bittet den Patienten um etwas Geduld, weil es sehr voll ist.

Nach ca. 20 Minuten begleitet die MFA den Patienten ins Arztzimmer und gibt die Versichertenkarte zurück.

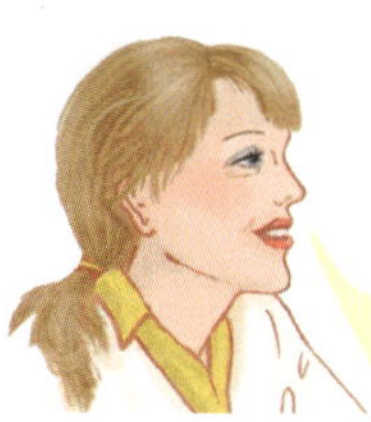

After the consultation

(The doctor took an X-ray, the ankle is not broken. Mr. Amin is sitting on the treatment couch.)

MFA erklärt Patient, dass sie einen Verband anlegen wird, um dem Knöchel zu stabilisieren und um die Schwellung gering zu halten.

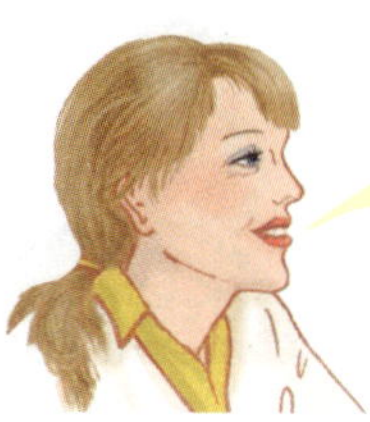

Patient fragt, was er machen soll.

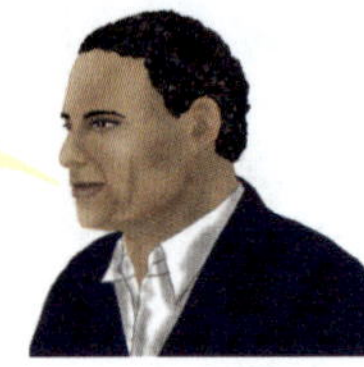

MFA sagt, dass der linke Fuß über den Rand der Liege platziert werden soll. Er soll den Fuß im rechten Winkel halten, während die MFA den Verband wickelt. Zunächst gibt die MFA zur besseren Heilung etwas Salbe auf den Knöchel. Dann fragt sie den Patienten, ob er die gelbe, pinke oder blaue Bandage bevorzugt.

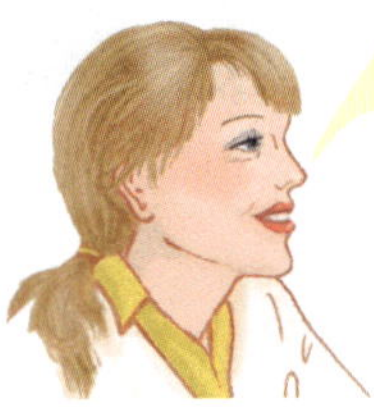

Patient mag die Farbe blau am liebsten und fragt, ob er den Fuß richtig hält.

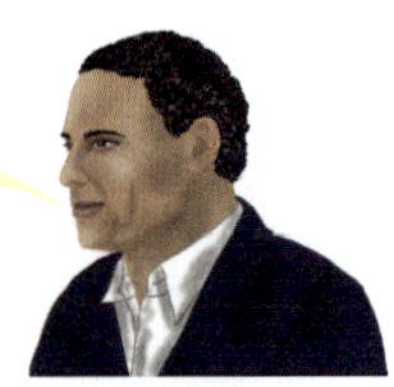

Die Fußposition ist gut. MFA beginnt an den Zehen und rollt den Verband bis über die Knöchel. MFA fragt Patient, ob der Verband zu stramm ist. Die Durchblutung muss noch o.k. sein.

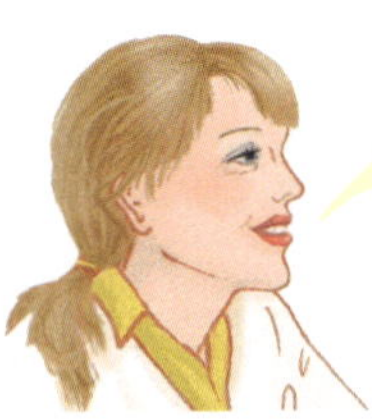

Patient sagt, dass der Verband sich gut anfühlt.

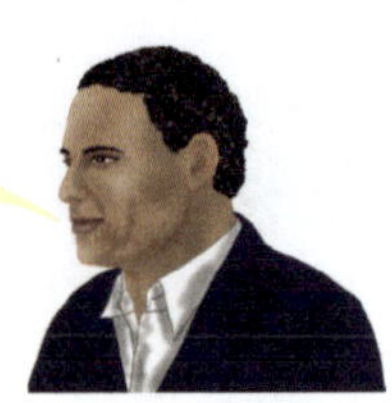

MFA stellt Verband fertig und erklärt dem Patienten, dass er ihn etwa 2 Tage tragen soll und sich dann wieder beim Doktor vorstellen muss. Sie rät dem Patienten, am besten vormittags zu kommen, weil die Praxis dann nicht so voll ist. Wenn der Verband zu stramm ist, soll er sich melden.

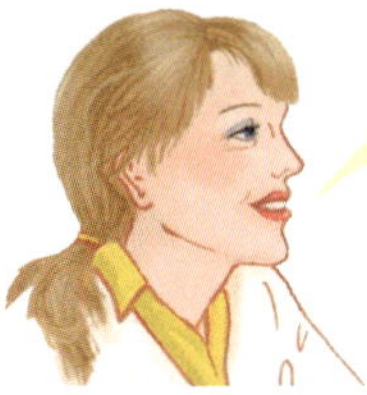

Patient benötigt eine AU, da er in seinem Restaurantjob viel stehen und laufen muss. Er fragt, ob er ein Schmerzmittel einnehmen kann, falls der Schmerz zu stark ist. Er fragt auch, ob er mit dem Verband duschen darf.

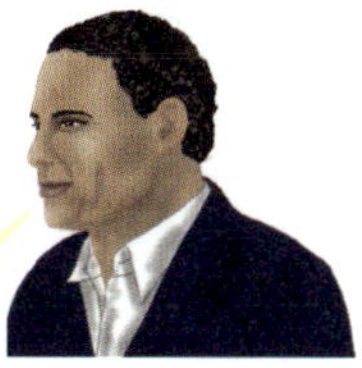

MFA sagt, dass Patient eine Plastiktüte um den Fuß tun kann, damit er nicht nass wird. MFA bittet den Patienten noch kurz zu warten, damit sie die AU ausdrucken und vom Arzt unterschreiben lassen kann. Sie wird den Arzt nach einem Schmerzmittel fragen.

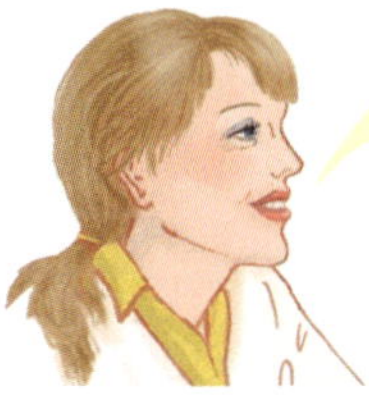

MFA übergibt die AU und bittet ihn, ein Formular an seinen Arbeitgeber und das andere an seine Krankenkasse zu schicken. MFA richtet vom Doktor aus, dass er entweder Aspirin oder Ibuprofen nehmen kann. Beide haben eine schmerzlindernde, entzündungshemmende und abschwellende Wirkung und sind frei verkäuflich in der Apotheke erhältlich.

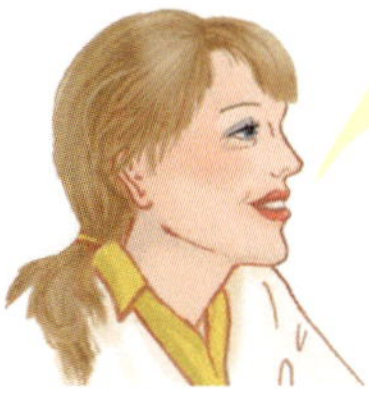

Patient sagt, dass er Ibuprofen zu Hause hat, da er es hin und wieder bei Kopfschmerzen einnimmt.

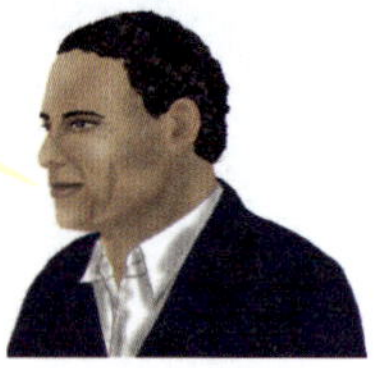

MFA weist den Patienten an, dass er den Knöchel gut mit einem Eispack kühlen soll – sie erklärt, wie häufig und wie lange. Er soll den Fuß so häufig wie möglich hochlegen und ihm Ruhe gönnen.

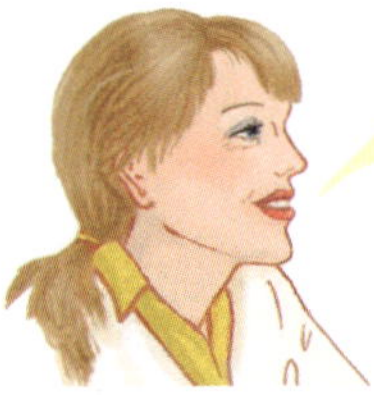

Patient fragt, ob er in die Sauna gehen darf.

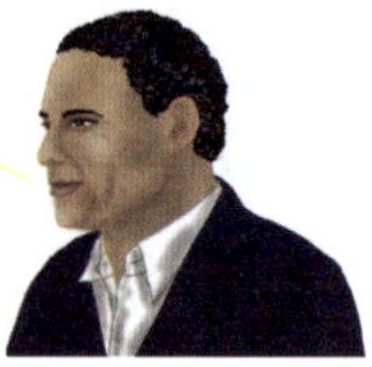

MFA beantwortet die Frage.

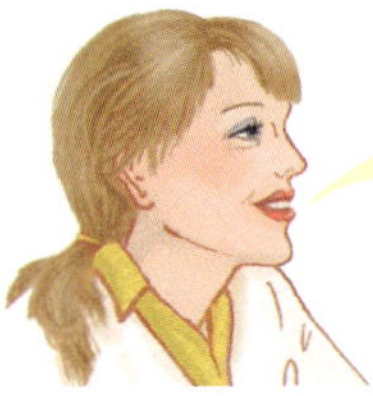

Patient bedankt und verabschiedet sich.

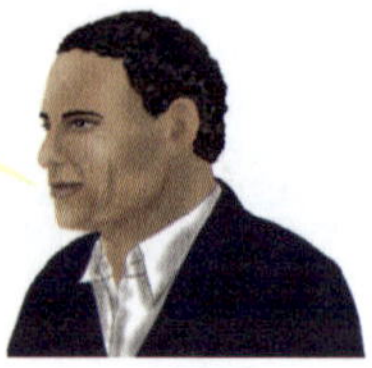

MFA wünscht gute Besserung.

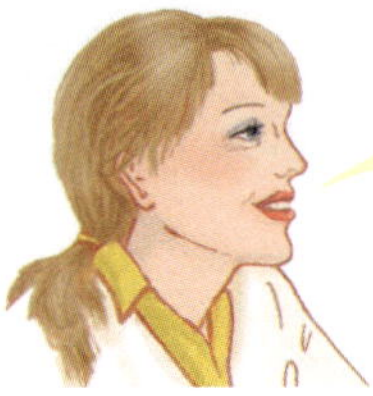

Ankle Sprain WORD SEARCH

6 **Can you find 24 hidden words? Find the hidden message in the remaining letters:**

A	P	E	X	E	R	C	I	S	E	P	P	A	Y	T
N	H	H	N	O	I	T	A	M	M	A	L	F	N	I
K	E	P	Y	T	S	I	W	T	C	I	Y	I	B	N
L	R	I	C	S	E	A	N	D	R	N	R	C	R	O
E	A	V	J	O	I	N	T	O	U	K	E	E	U	I
W	O	L	F	D	O	O	L	B	T	I	G	P	I	S
I	G	E	L	E	V	A	T	E	C	L	R	A	S	S
E	N	D	F	H	L	A	R	H	H	L	U	C	E	E
S	I	S	P	R	A	I	N	M	E	E	S	K	D	R
A	L	V	I	A	A	M	G	N	S	R	M	Y	P	P
E	L	A	S	T	I	C	B	A	N	D	A	G	E	M
R	E	C	I	V	D	A	T	V	M	X	A	P	N	O
C	W	V	B	L	D	E	C	U	D	E	R	U	Y	C
N	S	D	E	R	U	J	N	I	R	Z	N	N	O	L
I	B	L	E	E	D	I	N	G	H	E	Z	T	H	O

....

....

....

....

....

....

....

....

Hidden message: ....

5 Getting an X-ray

LISTENING Track 6

1 **Listen to the dialog and answer the following questions:**

- *What examination is being performed?*
- *What instructions does the medical assistant give?*

READING

2 **Read the following text and find the German words 3. Check any other new vocabulary in the vocabulary list or in a dictionary.**

tissue, muscles, radiographs, osteoarthritis, lead aprons

gray = AE, grey = BE

1 to emit – aussenden
2 captured – eingefangen
3 gap – spalt
4 likelihood – Wahrscheinlichkeit
5 exposure – Bestrahlung

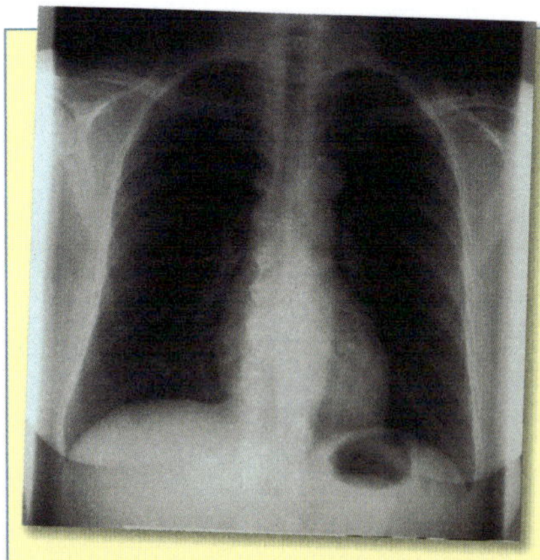

X-rays are a type of high energy radiation. They pass easily through the soft tissues of the body. The denser the tissue, the fewer the X-rays that can pass through it. The X-ray machine emits[1] X-rays which pass through your body. The X-rays are captured[2] on a film which is then developed. The more X-rays absorbed by the film, the blacker it is when developed. Therefore, dense parts of the body such as bones that block many of the X-rays show up white. Hollow parts of the body such as parts of the lung show up black. Soft tissues such as organs and muscles show up as various shades of gray. X-ray images (radiographs) can show teeth, bone fractures and other abnormalities of bone as well as gaps[3] in joints and some joint abnormalities such as osteoarthritis. They also show the size and shape of the heart and changes in the density of some softer tissues. For example, a lung or breast tumor shows up as a shadow on a chest or breast X-ray because it is denser than an air-filled lung or normal breast tissue.

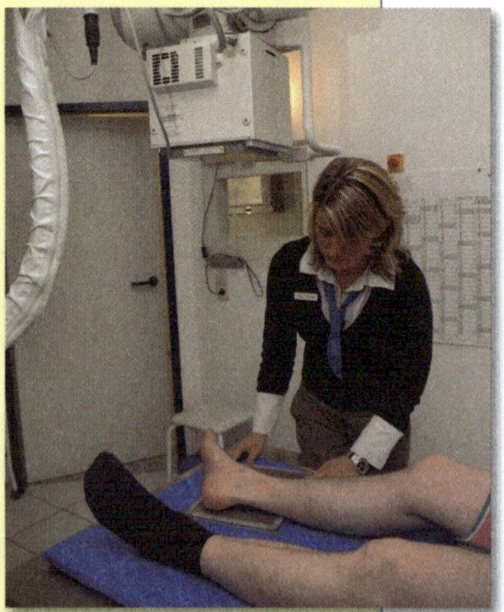

An X-ray is a quick, easy, cheap and painless test. You cannot see or feel X-rays. When having an X-ray, you need to take off some clothes, all your jewellry, your watch and glasses because metal gets in the way of taking a clear picture. You will be asked to sit or lie on a table or stand beside the X-ray machine. The medical assistant will help you to get into the right position. You should hold very still while the X-ray is being taken to get a clear picture. You may also have to hold your breath. After a short moment, you can move again. Often you will have to change position to get another image from a different perspective. When it is all done you can get dressed again.

There is little risk with having one X-ray test. However, with repeated tests the likelihood[4] of body cells being damaged by the radiation grows, possibly leading to cancer in the future. The dose of X-ray radiation needed to get a good image is always kept to the minimum. Staff taking the X-ray images always wear lead aprons or go behind a protective screen during the exposure[5]. Patients too, have to be shielded with lead aprons. They should also have an X-ray record card and show it to the medical staff to avoid having repeated radiographs.
If at all possible, pregnant women should not have radiographs taken because there is a small risk that X-rays may cause an abnormality to the unborn child. This is why women always have to be asked if they are, or might be pregnant before having an X-ray.

COMPREHENSION

3 **Find the following words in the text:**

Röntgenstrahlen | Strahlung | dicht, Dichte | weiches Gewebe
Röntgenpass | entwickeln | hohl | Röntgenbild | Grautöne
Gelenkspalt | Knochenbruch | Größe und Form | Schatten
schmerzlos | medizinisches Personal | Geschwulst
Doppelaufnahme | Schmuck | Uhr | ruhig | Brille
bewegen | sich anziehen | beschädigt | Krebs | Bleischürze
Schwangere | Schutzscheibe | Blickwinkel

4 **Match the sentence parts:**

1. X-rays pass easily
2. The less dense the body tissue
3. Dense tissue like bone
4. X-ray images can detect
5. Body organs and muscles

a. the darker the X-ray image becomes.
b. changes in lung or breast tissue
c. show up in different shades of gray.
d. through the soft tissues of the body.
e. blocks X-rays and the film shows up white.

5 **Correct the false statements:**

1. Taking an X-ray image hurts.

....

2. The patient has to undress completely but can leave in earrings and piercings and leave on bracelets, necklaces and glasses.

....

3. The patient can move while the X-ray image is taken.

....

4. The doctor always needs just one X-ray image.

....

....

5. Protection is not necessary as X-ray radiation is harmless.

....

....

....

....

6. It is not risky to X-ray pregnant women.

....

....

....

DIALOG / ROLEPLAY

6 **Write a dialog with a partner. Complete the speech bubbles:**

Since this morning Mrs. O'Neill has had a terrible backache. She can hardly move and is not able to bend her back at all. Her husband has just driven her to the orthopedist. Now they are entering the doctor's practice. Mrs. O'Neill's face shows she is in pain:

MFA grüßt und bietet Hilfe an.

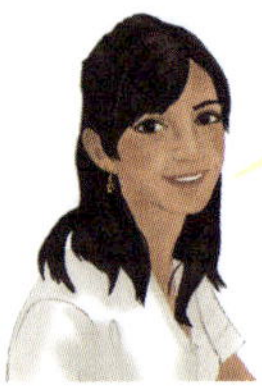

Mr. O'Neill berichtet, was mit seiner Frau los ist. Sie kommen als Notfall und möchten zum Arzt.

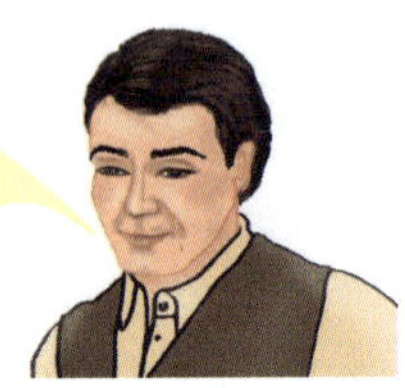

MFA bestätigt, dass sie zum Arzt kann und fragt, ob die Patientin in der Zwischenzeit im Wartezimmer sitzen kann oder lieber liegen möchte.

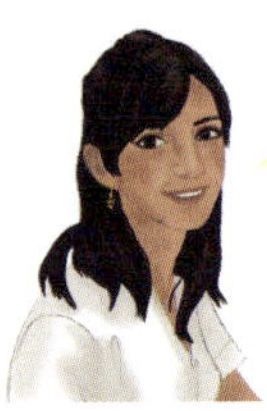

Patientin meint, dass sie kann im Wartezimmer sitzen kann.

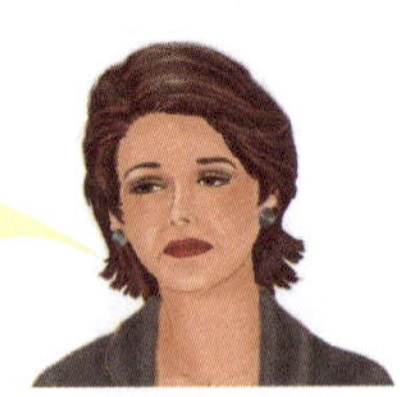

MFA bittet um die KVK, schickt das Ehepaar ins Wartezimmer und bittet um etwas Geduld, da es sehr voll ist. Sie wird dann aufgerufen.

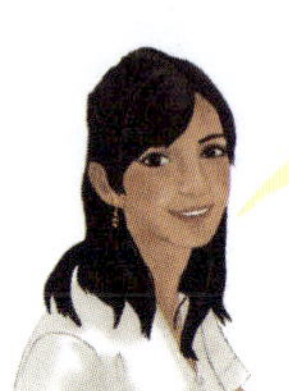

20 minutes later

MFA ruft Patientin auf und begleitet sie ins Behandlungszimmer. Sie gibt die KVK ihrem Mann.

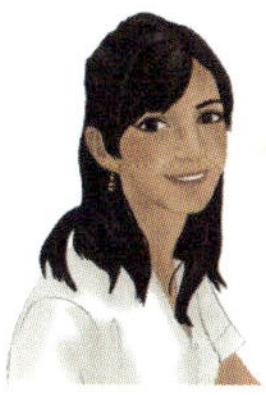

After the consultation

The doctor has examined Mrs. O'Neill. He asks the medical assistant to take X-rays of the patient's back:

MFA fragt nach möglicher Schwangerschaft.

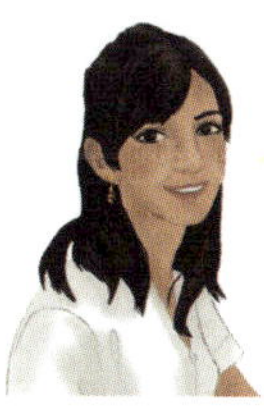

Patientin verneint mit Sicherheit.

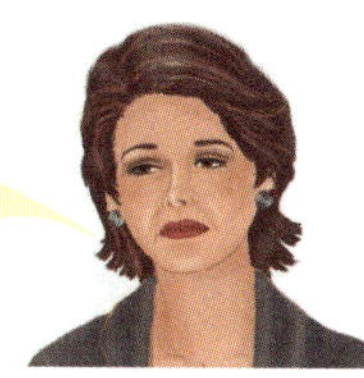

MFA bittet Patientin, ihr zum Röntgen zu folgen. Dort angekommen, bittet sie die Patientin ihren Oberkörper freizumachen, die Hose auszuziehen und Kette, Ohrringe und Uhr in der Kabine abzulegen. Sie wird sie dann reinholen.

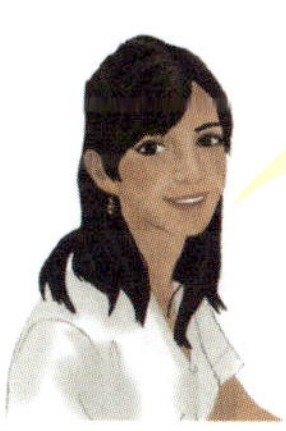

Patientin fragt, ob sie auch den BH ausziehen muss.

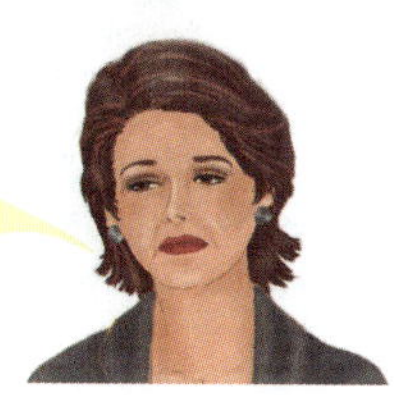

MFA bejaht, da das Metall im BH die Aufnahme stören würde.

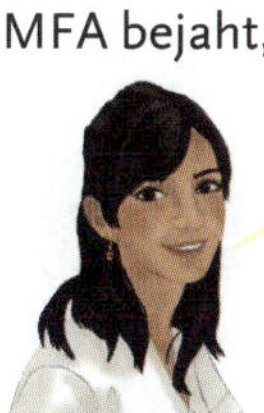

5 minutes later (her husband helped her to get undressed)

MFA bittet Patientin, sich auf den Tisch zu legen, auf den Rücken. Nachdem sie alles eingestellt hat, bittet sie die Patientin ganz ruhig liegen zu bleiben und den Atem kurz anzuhalten, während sie die Aufnahme macht. Hinter der Schutzscheibe fordert sie die Patientin nochmals auf, nicht zu atmen und löst aus. Dann teilt sie der Patientin mit, dass sie weiteratmen kann.

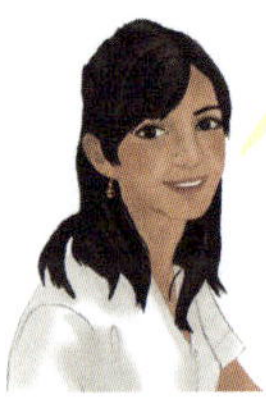

....

....

....

....

....

MFA geht wieder zur Patientin und bittet sie, sich für eine weitere Aufnahme auf die rechte Seite zu legen und die Beine zu strecken.
Sie fordert die Patientin erneut auf, sich nicht zu bewegen und nicht zu atmen.

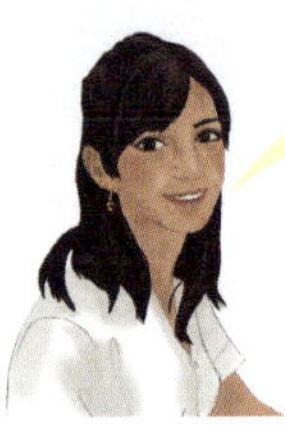

....

....

....

....

MFA teilt mit, dass sie jetzt noch eine Aufnahme nur von der Halswirbelsäule macht. Patientin soll sich wieder auf den Rücken legen. Sie bedeckt das Genital der Patientin zum Schutz mit einer Bleischürze und gibt wieder ihre Anweisungen.
Dann teilt sie mit, dass die Patientin fertig ist, sich wieder bewegen und sich wieder anziehen kann.

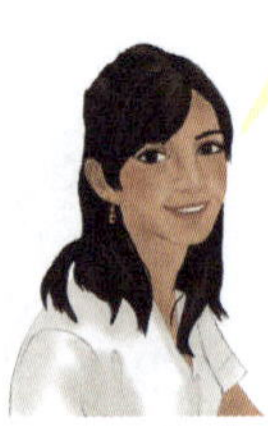

....

....

....

....

....

....

Patientin bittet MFA, ihr hoch zu helfen, da sie Schmerzen hat.

....

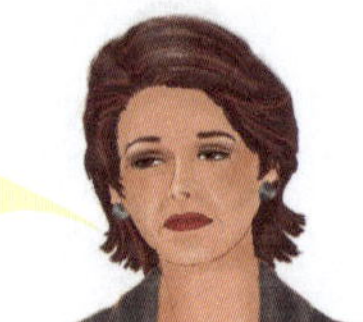

MFA bittet ihren Mann zur Hilfe, der draußen gewartet hat und teilt der Patientin mit, dass sie wieder im Wartezimmer Platz nehmen soll. Sie entwickelt jetzt die Röntgenaufnahmen und der Arzt wird diese dann mit ihr besprechen. Sie verabschiedet sich und wünscht gute Besserung.

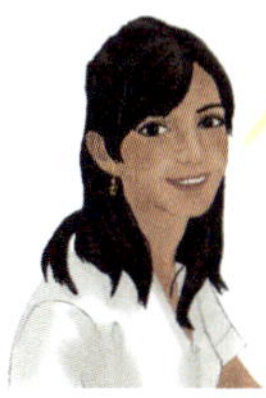

Patientin bedankt und verabschiedet sich.

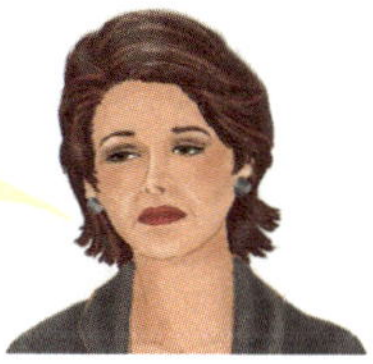

X-ray WORD SEARCH

7 Can you find 31 hidden words? Find the hidden message in the remaining letters:

```
D C E R T S H A D O W S J S K
N R H U O N R O B N U S E T S
T E A A S M A T A M M E W R I
N E C C N S U N K O L L E E R
I E E K D G I T G V I N L T A
O O F T L R I T T E F I L C D
J F Y O H A O N T S R A R H I
E G A M A D C C G F A P Y E A
F R A C T U R E E R O E A S T
N O R P A D A E L R O S R T I
N O I T I S O P S U Y O B B O
S G N I R R A E R S B A M R N
P O L E V E D T R A E H R A C
E S E S S A L G B E N D L X E
Y T I S N E D S S U C S I D T
```

Hidden message: ....

6 Automatic Blood Pressure Measurement (ABPM)

LISTENING Track 7

1 **Listen to the dialog and answer the following questions:**

- *Why is Mr. Pressure at the doctor's practice?*
- *What does the medical assistant do?*

READING

2 **Read the following text and find the German words 3. Check any other new vocabulary in the vocabulary list or in a dictionary.**

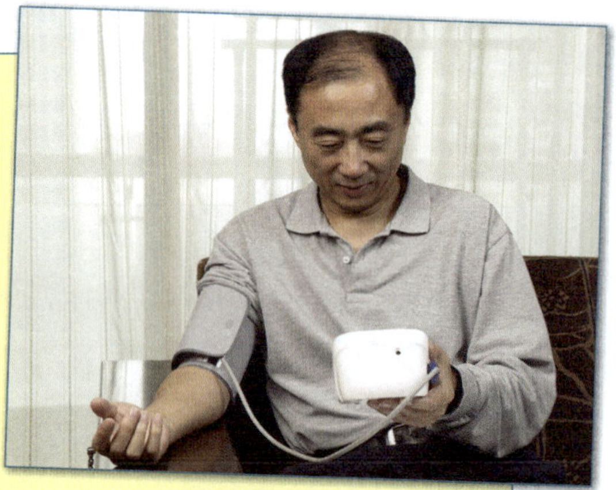

ABPM – Automatic Blood Pressure Measurement – Langzeitblutdruck

MA: Good morning.
PAT: Good morning, I have an appointment. My name is Mr. Pressure.
MA: OK, fine Mr. Pressure. Take a seat in the waiting-room for a minute please.
PAT: OK.

Some minutes later...

MA: Mr. Pressure, could you come through please? Room number 3.

In the treatment room: Mr. Pressure is getting a blood pressure machine fixed because his blood pressure is too high. He has to wear it for 24 hours.

MA: Please take off your T-shirt.
PAT: OK.
MA: Now I'm going to wrap the cuff around your arm. Could you stretch your arm out, please?

The medical assistant is putting on the cuff...

MA: Okay, now I'm going to fasten the belt above your hip and attach it to the computer. Does everything fit OK? Nothing too tight?
PAT: Could you loosen the belt a little bit?
MA: Yes, of course...
And now I'm just going to connect the cuff with the computer. The first meausurement is just starting, please relax your arm.

The machine is pumping up, the first result is 155/95 mmHg

MA: Oh, that's a little too high Mr. Pressure.
PAT: Will I die???
MA: No, you won't, not today, not here... I'm only joking. Don't worry.
The machine measures four times an hour during the day and during the night it pumps up every 30 minutes. When the cuff starts pumping up relax your arm. Don't take a shower or bath with the machine. Write down everything you do during the day. Tomorrow at the same time you can take off the machine and bring it back here.
PAT: OK, thank you very much. See you tomorrow. Have a nice day, bye bye.
MA: Bye Mr. Pressure, same to you.

COMPREHENSION

3 **Try to say it in English:**

Hallo Mr. Pressure, bitte nehmen Sie noch im Wartezimmer Platz.

....

Bitte ziehen Sie ihr T-Shirt aus, Mr. Pressure.

....

Ich werde jetzt den Computer und die Manschette miteinander verbinden.

....

Die Maschine misst viermal in der Stunde am Tag, und in der Nacht wird sie alle halbe Stunde messen.

....

....

Schreiben Sie auf, was Sie den Tag über tun.

....

4 **Fill in the gaps:**

appointment – bath – belt – 2x cuff – computer – going to – relax – shower – stretch out

I have an .... at 10 a.m.

Now I'm .... put on the cuff. Please stretch out your arm.

I am going to fasten the ....

I am going to connect the .... with the ....

The measurement is starting, please .... your arm.

Don't take a .... or .... with the machine.

ABPM WORD SEARCH

5 **Can you find the 12 words in this square?**

appointmenthsmkxoansbxzsmalwaowwlsjend
jksbagqsjcusbsndcjcshowernskdndidshwkwbj
sownducbjmdivcnejfcndesidsmjugohjlskwsixjs
ndendiwmekemdsdmsjcnmddkdfasteneonxoya
ndbeltlcjendodmdjchkanxusloyshjfdorbloodqpr
essurejxuwbfcichsmdxochlsosnebejfbdkssineb
ekxilxidscomputerhsosheifbdndciemdodjerelax
msossiduwbenfcjbakalaspieneknbathlshnudbd
mdicmwaitingzroomsmdisnskxjwnsixnskcidnwn
medicalzassistantnsmskisnskpatientmjnsosnwj
cwjewndkcxhwbwjwwiwkxndenenejcuffncldndid
nendkciendnddkhso

1 .... 7 ....

2 .... 8 ....

3 .... 9 ....

4 .... 10 ....

5 .... 11 ....

6 .... 12 ....

6 **Try to make three or four sentences for the words above:**

....

....

....

....

....

....

....

....

....

....

DIALOG / ROLEPLAY

7 **Write a dialog with a partner. Complete the speech bubbles:**

MFA begrüßt den Patienten.

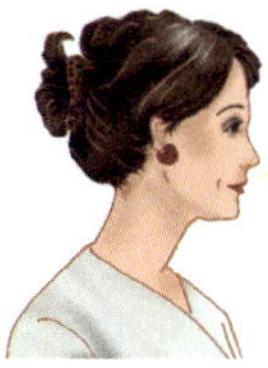

Patient hat einen Termin.

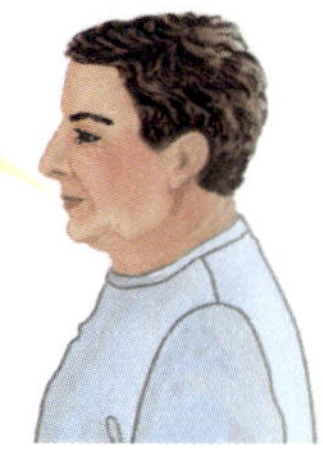

MFA bittet den Patienten, einen Augenblick im Wartezimmer Platz zu nehmen.

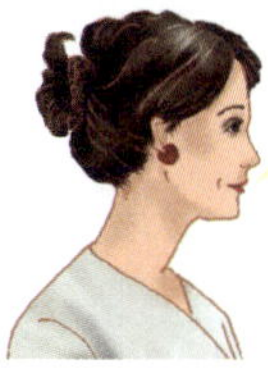

Patient willigt ein und setzt sich in das Wartezimmer.

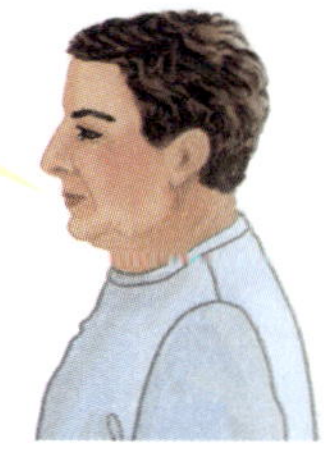

MFA ruft den Patienten auf und bittet ihn, in Raum 3 zu gehen.

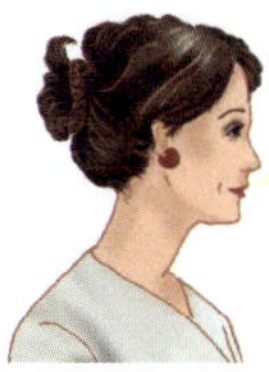

MFA bittet den Patienten, sein T-Shirt auszuziehen.

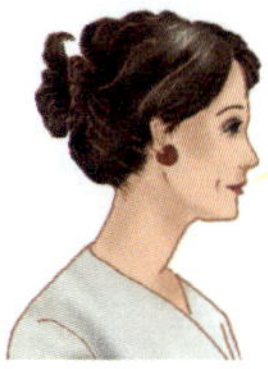

Patient willigt ein und zieht sein T- Shirt aus.

....

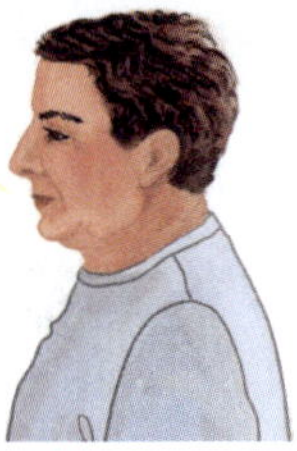

MFA erklärt, dass sie jetzt die Blutdruckmanschette anlegt und er dafür bitte den Arm ausstrecken soll.

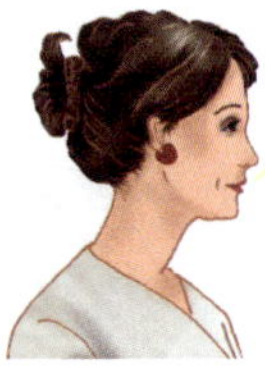

....

....

MFA legt den Gürtel um seine Hüfte und befestigt das Gerät am Gürtel. Sie fragt ihn, ob alles bequem sitzt.

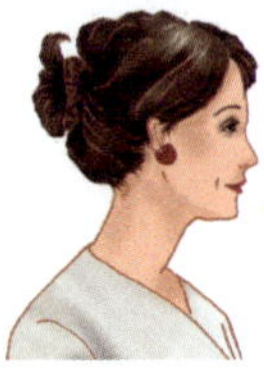

....

....

....

Patient bittet, den Gürtel etwas lockerer zu machen.

....

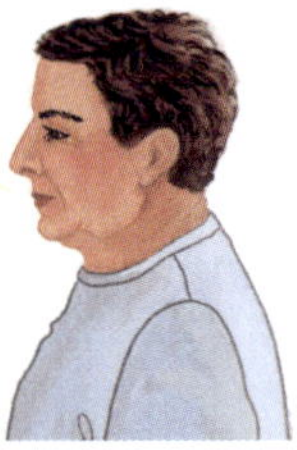

MFA willigt ein und verbindet dann das Gerät mit der Manschette. Sie weist darauf hin, dass jetzt die erste Messung startest und er bitte seinen Arm locker halten soll.

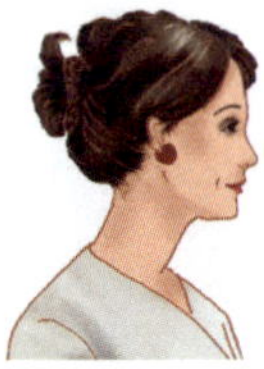

....

....

....

....

....

MFA bemerkt, dass der Wert etwas zu hoch ist.

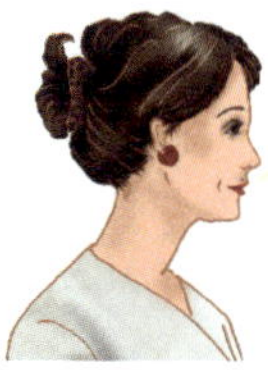

Patient ist verängstigt und fragt, ob er jetzt sterben muss.

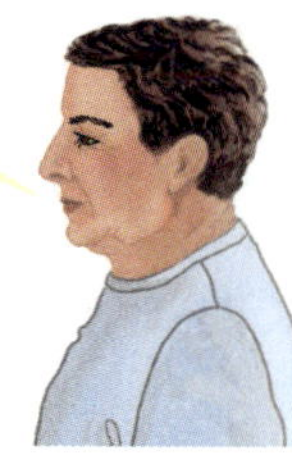

MFA beruhigt ihn und sagt, dass er nicht sterben muss. Sie erklärt ihm, dass das Gerät am Tag alle 15 Minuten und in der Nacht alle 30 Minuten messen wird. Patient soll den Arm während der Messungen ruhig halten. Er darf nicht baden oder duschen mit dem Gerät. Er soll alles aufschreiben, was er den Tag über tut. Morgen um die gleiche Zeit soll der Patient das Gerät abnehmen und in der Praxis abgeben.

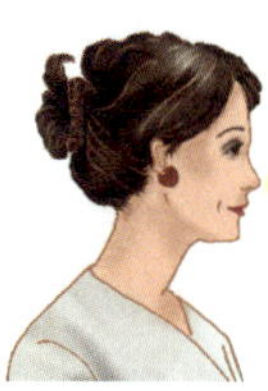

Patient stimmt zu, bedankt sich, wünscht einen schönen Tag und sagt, dass sie sich morgen wieder sehen.

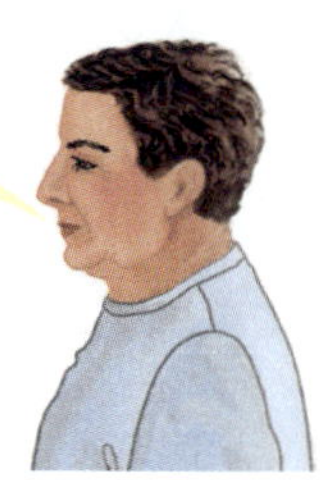

MFA verabschiedet sich ebenfalls.

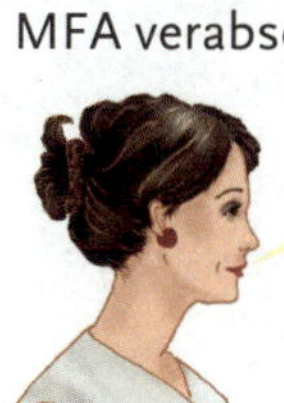

7 Electrocardiography (ECG)

LISTENING Track 8

1 **Listen to the dialog and answer the following questions:**

- *Which examination is being performed?*
- *What instructions does the medical assistant give?*

READING

2 **Read the text and check the vocabulary in bold print in the word list or in a dictionary:**

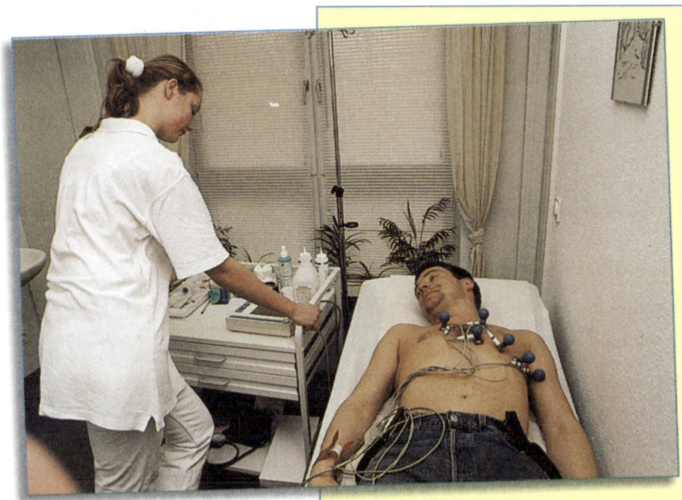

What is an electrocardiogram?

An electrocardiogram (ECG) **records** the electrical activity of the heart. The heart produces electrical impulses which spread[1] through the heart muscle to make the heart **contract**. These impulses can be **detected** by the ECG machine. The electrocardiogram is used to detect abnormal heart rhythms. You may have an ECG to help find the **cause** of symptoms such as palpitations[2] or **chest pain**. Sometimes it is done as part of routine tests, for example, before you have an operation.

The ECG test is **painless** and **harmless**. The ECG machine records electrical impulses coming from your body – it does not put any electricity into your body.

How is it done?

First **personal data** of the patient including current[3] **medication** have to be entered into the ECG-computer. Then small metal electrodes are stuck onto your arms, legs and chest. Wires[4] from the **electrodes** are connected to the ECG machine. The machine detects and amplifies[5] the electrical impulses that **occur** with each heartbeat and records them onto a paper or computer. A few heartbeats are recorded from different sets of electrodes. The test takes about five minutes. The patient is asked to take off his pullover and shirt and **remove** any clothing from the lower legs. Metal **watches** also have to be removed. Then the patient has to lie down on the **treatment table**. Gel or spray is used to help place the electrodes. Sometimes **thick chest hair** has to be shaved to allow the electrodes to be placed. The patient **must not** speak or move during the examination. If the patient feels cold, this can also **falsify** the **results**. A warm room temperature or **blanket** should stop the patient feeling too cold.

electrocardiogram,
muscle,
palpitations,
electrodes,
coronary

What does an ECG show?

The electrodes on the different parts of the body detect electrical impulses coming from different directions within the heart. There are normal patterns[6] for each electrode. Many heart **disorders** produce abnormal patterns. The heart disorders that can be detected include:

- abnormal **heart rhythms**; if the heart rate is very fast, very slow, or irregular
- a **heart attack**, and if it was recent[7] or some time ago. A heart attack causes **damage** to the heart muscle, and heals with scar tissue[8]. These can be detected by abnormal ECG patterns.
- an **enlarged** heart; this causes stronger impulses than normal.

However, an ECG cannot detect **coronary heart disease**.

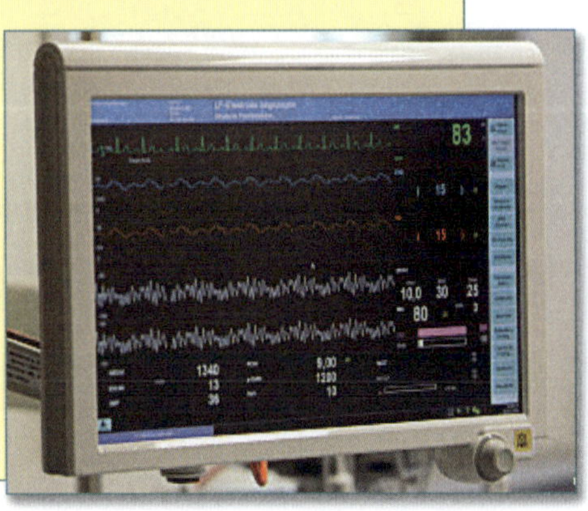

1 to spread – ausbreiten
2 palpitations – Herzklopfen
3 current – derzeitig
4 wire – Kabel
5 to amplify – verstärken
6 pattern – Muster
7 recent – kürzlich, vor kurzem
8 scar tissue – Narbengewebe

VOCABULARY

3 **Label the picture with the following words:**

examination table – ECG – electrodes – chest – wrist – ankles – wire – patient

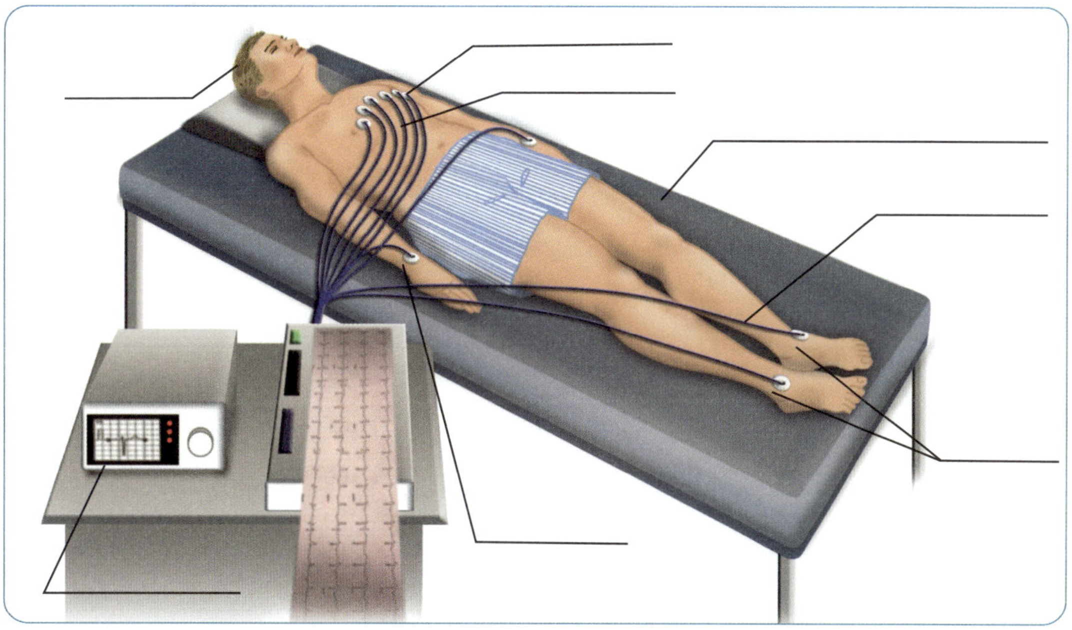

COMPREHENSION

4 **ECG Criss-Cross**

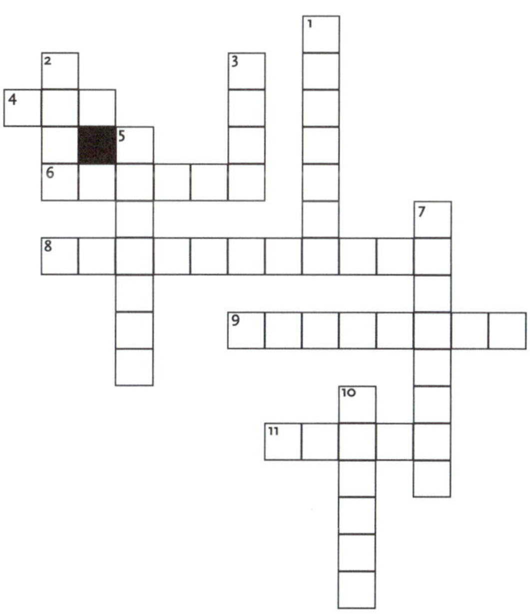

Across

4. electrocardiogram
6. to take off/away
8. heart beats fast with irregular rhythm
9. to become shorter and smaller
11. to cut hair from body

Down

1. something to keep you warm
2. mark on the skin after a wound has healed
3. cable
5. to increase in intensity
7. bigger than normal
10. physical harm

5 **True or false? Correct false sentences:**

	T/F
1. An ECG detects electrical impulses from the heart.	
2. An ECG can diagnose brain activity.	
3. An ECG is harmless because it puts electricity into your body.	
4. ECG electrodes are stuck onto your arms, legs and back.	
5. The test takes about five minutes.	
6. The patient sits on the treatment table during the examination.	
7. The patient has to take off all his clothes.	
8. If a man has thick chest hair you have to shave it.	
9. Spray or gel is used to improve the contact between skin and electrodes.	
10. During the examination the patient is allowed to speak.	
11. If the patient is cold you can offer him/her a blanket.	
12. An ECG can diagnose an irregular heart rhythm, heart attacks and enlarged hearts.	

DIALOG / ROLE PLAY

6 **Write a dialog with a partner. Complete the speech bubbles:**

MFA begrüßt die Patientin.

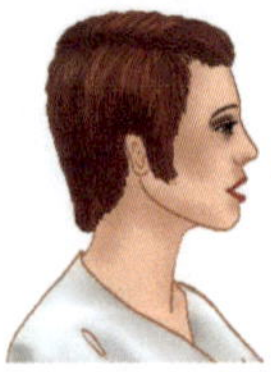

Patientin hat einen Termin um 9:15 Uhr zum EKG.

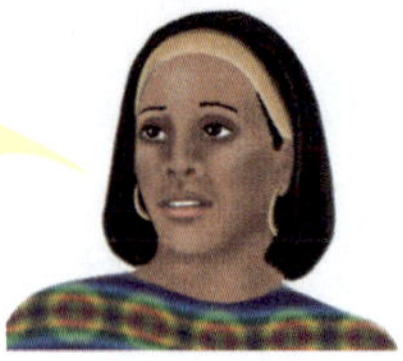

MFA bittet um die Versichertenkarte und den Überweisungsschein vom Hausarzt. Nachdem sie die Patientendaten eingelesen hat, bittet sie die Patientin, direkt im EKG Zimmer Platz zu nehmen. Dieses befindet sich auf dem Flur, dritte Tür rechts neben dem Labor. MFA sagt, dass sie sofort kommt, um das EKG zu schreiben.

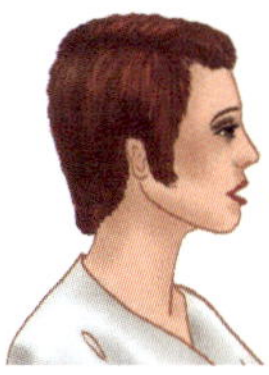

Im EKG Zimmer erklärt die MFA der Patientin, dass sie jetzt ein EKG schreibt und warum. Dazu soll Patientin den Oberkörper frei machen, Schuhe und Socken ausziehen und die Uhr ablegen.

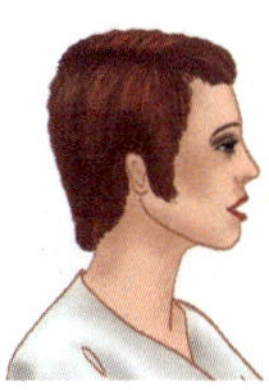

Patientin sagt, dass sie heute eine Strumpfhose trägt und fragt nach, ob sie diese wirklich ausziehen muss. Sie fragt, ob Sie auch den BH ausziehen muss.

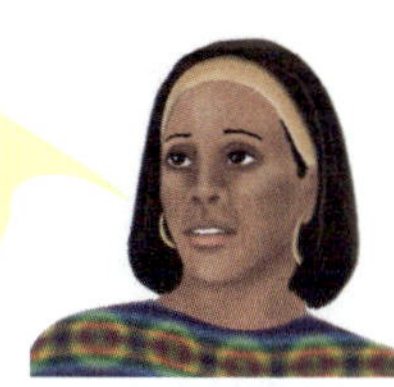

MFA erklärt, dass das notwendig ist, damit sie das EKG korrekt anlegen kann. Die Patientin soll sich auf die Liege legen. Die MFA erklärt, dass und wo Elektroden befestigt werden. Durch das Elektrodenspray kann es etwas kalt werden .

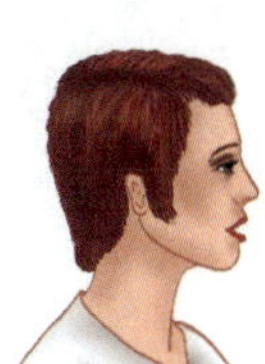

Patientin ängstigt das etwas, da sie sich fragt, ob sie einen Stromschlag bekommen kann. Patientin möchte auch gerne wissen, ob diese Untersuchung schmerzhaft ist.

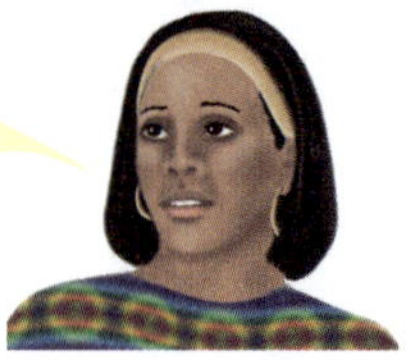

MFA beruhigt die Patientin, indem sie ihr mitteilt, dass kein Strom in den Körper fließt, sondern die Herzströme der Patientin aufgezeichnet werden. Außerdem ist diese Untersuchung nicht schmerzhaft.

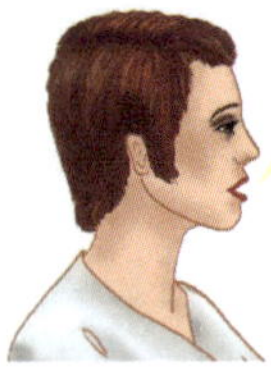

Patientin äußert, dass ihr etwas kalt ist.

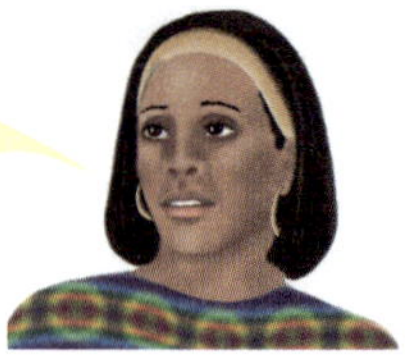

MFA gibt der Patientin eine Decke und dreht die Heizung höher. MFA fordert Patientin auf, normal zu atmen, sich nicht zu bewegen und nicht zu sprechen.

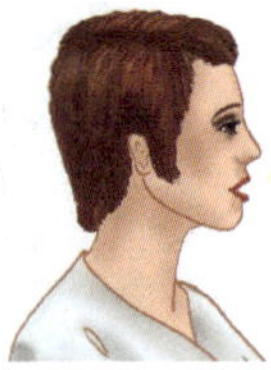

Patientin fragt nach der Aufzeichnung, ob ihr Herz gesund ist.

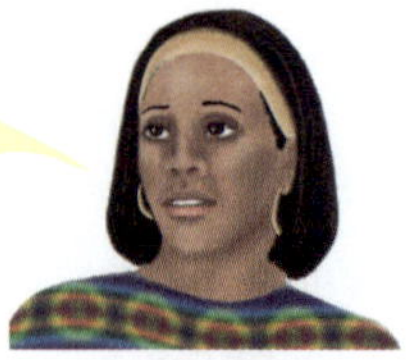

MFA weist Patientin darauf hin, dass das der Arzt mit ihr besprechen wird. Sie reicht Papier, um das Elektrodenspray abzuwischen und teilt mit, dass die Patientin sich wieder anziehen kann. MFA bittet Patientin, noch kurz im Wartezimmer Platz zu nehmen, bis sie aufgerufen wird. MFA verabschiedet sich und wünscht einen schönen Tag

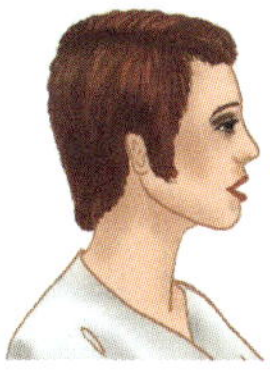

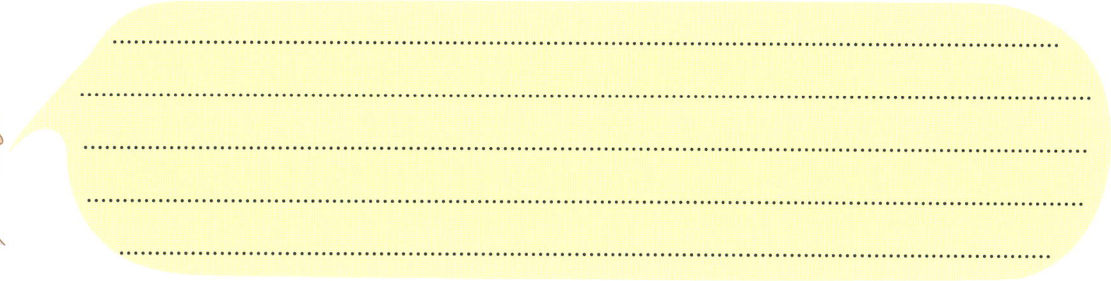

7 **Write a dialog using the role cards below: (For advanced students)**

MFA	**Patient, männlich, 43 Jahre**
– Begrüßung. Versicherungskarte. – Das EKG Zimmer ist am Ende des Flurs rechts. – Informieren Sie den Patienten über die Untersuchung. – Bitten Sie den Patienten, die erforderlichen Kleidungsstücke auszuziehen und sich auf die Behandlungsliege zu legen. – Nehmen Sie die Patientendaten auf. – Erklären Sie, was Sie tun. – Der Patient hat dichtes Brusthaar. – Sie benötigen Elektrodenspray. – Fordern Sie den Patienten auf, nicht zu sprechen, sich nicht zu bewegen und normal zu atmen. – Fragen Sie den Patienten, ob alles o.k. ist. – Reagieren Sie auf den Patienten. – Bitten Sie ihn, nach der Untersuchung im Sprechzimmer des Doktors Platz zu nehmen.	– Sie haben einen Termin zum EKG um 10:45. – Beim Ausziehen fragen Sie, ob Sie auch Ihre Rolex und Goldkette ablegen müssen. – Sie möchten wissen, ob die Untersuchung wegen des Stroms gefährlich ist. – Sie sind nicht begeistert, dass die MFA Ihr Brusthaar rasieren möchte. – Ihnen ist während der Messung etwas kalt. – Sie müssen auf einmal während der Untersuchung husten. – Nach der Untersuchung fragen Sie die MFA, ob Ihr Herz gesund ist.

Exercise ECG (ECG Stress Test, Stress Echocardiogram)

VOCABULARY

8 **Label the picture with as many words as you can:**

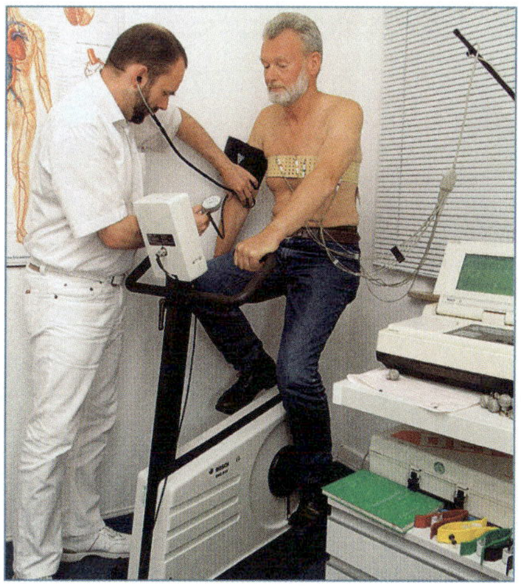

READING

9 Read the text and check the vocabulary in the word list or with a dictionary:

coronary, electrodes

1 severity – Schweregrad
2 resting ECG – Ruhe-EKG
3 treadmill – Laufband
4 half way through – nach der Hälfte
5 further – weiter
6 degree of difficulty – Schwierigkeitsgrad
7 either... or – entweder... oder
8 to monitor – überwachen
9 at least – mindestens
10 recommended – empfohlen

A ECG stress test helps to diagnose the cause of the patient's heart trouble and the severity[1] of coronary heart disease. The patient will be asked about the medication he/she is on and if he/she feels physically able to take the test.
First, a resting ECG[2] is carried out. The blood pressure and the pulse rate are measured as well. The ECG results are handed to the doctor and the exercise ECG cannot be started until the doctor gives his OK. Electrodes are placed on the patient's chest.
An exercise-based ECG is carried out while the patient exercises on a bicycle (or treadmill[3]). The patient is asked to cycle for about two minutes starting with 50 watt. When halfway through[4], the blood pressure is measured and documented. With every further[5] measurement the degree of difficulty[6] is increased by 25 watts. This process will go on until either[7] the patient's maximum heart rate is reached or the patient says that he/she cannot go on any longer. It is important to monitor[8] the patient all along the process because the patient could become very short of breath or even collapse. In that case the test will be stopped to avoid the risk of a heart attack.
The test takes about 15 minutes. The patient should not eat a heavy meal for at least[9] one hour before the test. Loose fitting clothes and shoes are recommended[10].

COMPREHENSION

10 Match the sentence parts:

1. A stress test can diagnose
2. The medical assistant has to ask
3. Before the stress test
4. The doctor has to
5. A stress test is carried out
6. The cycling gets
7. The test is stopped

a. an ECG at rest is recorded.
b. on a treadmill or bicycle.
c. if the patient feels physically able to do the test.
d. gradually more difficult.
e. when the patient has severe difficulties breathing.
f. coronary heart disease.
g. approve the stress test.

11 True or false? Correct false sentences:

	T/F
1. Only a resting ECG can detect coronary heart disease.	
2. The medical assistant has to ask the patient if he/she takes heart medication.	
3. During the stress test vital signs are measured.	
4. The patient lies on the treatment table during the stress test.	
5. The physical difficulty is gradually increased during the test.	
6. During the test you can leave the patient alone because there are no risks for the patient.	
7. The stress test takes longer than an ECG at rest.	
8. The patient does not have to prepare for the test.	

DIALOG / ROLE PLAY

12 **Work with a partner, write a dialog between Mrs. Angina and you:**

Doctor Heartache suspects[11] that his 60-year-old patient Mrs. Angina suffers from coronary heart disease. Mrs. Angina is a little overweight and hardly exercises. Your boss instructs you to record an exercise ECG. You have written the ECG at rest:

11 to suspect – vermuten

MFA informiert die Patientin, dass jetzt ein Belastungs-EKG durchgeführt wird und bittet die Patientin, sich ihre Schuhe wieder anzuziehen und sich auf das Fahrrad zu setzen.

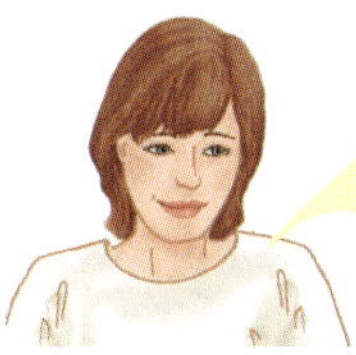

....

....

....

Die Patientin antwortet.

....

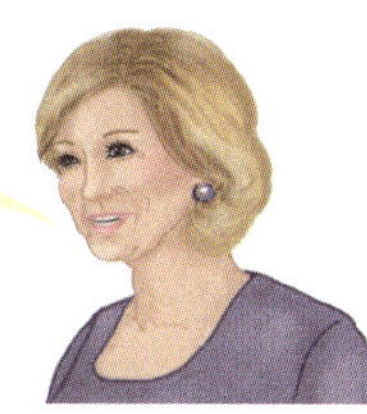

MFA legt die Elektroden und das Blutdruckmessgerät an und informiert die Patientin, dass das Gerät alle 2 Minuten den Blutdruck misst. Sie beginnt mit der 1. Messung und fragt Patientin, ob sie Sport treibt.

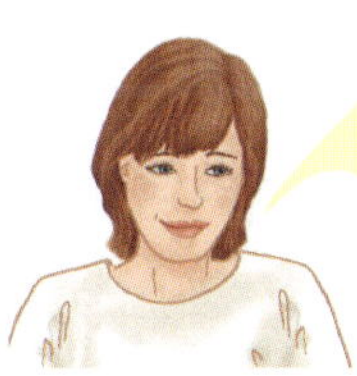

....

....

....

....

Die Patientin geht einmal die Woche schwimmen, sonst treibt sie keinen Sport.

....

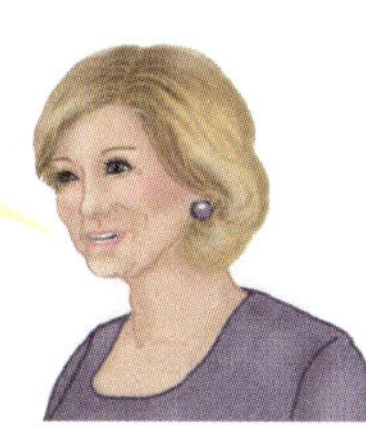

MFA erklärt der Patientin, dass sie treten muss, bis sie das grüne Licht sieht und diese Geschwindigkeit halten soll. Falls Probleme mit der Atmung, Schmerzen in der Brust oder den Beinen auftreten, soll sie Bescheid geben. MFA bittet die Patientin, zu beginnen.

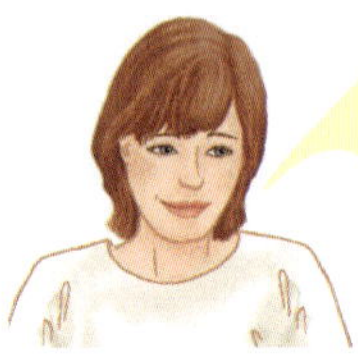

2 minutes later

MFA fragt die Patientin nach ihrem Befinden und teilt mit, dass es jetzt anstrengender wird zu treten. Die grüne Lampe soll weiterhin aufleuchten.

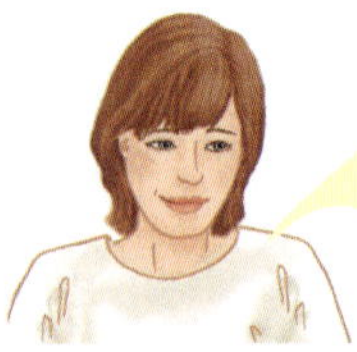

Die Patientin sagt, dass es anstrengend ist, es ihr aber gut geht.

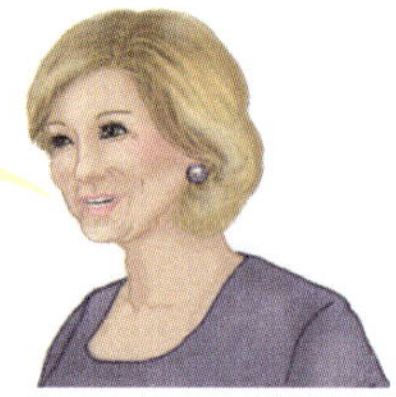

10 minutes later

Der Test ist beendet. MFA lobt die Patientin, entfernt die Elektroden, bietet der Patientin an, sich am Waschbecken frisch zu machen und fordert sie auf, sich wieder anzuziehen. Die Patientin soll sich dann direkt ins Sprechzimmer setzen.

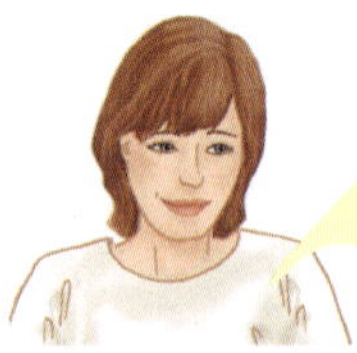

ECG WORD SEARCH

13 **Can you find 23 hidden words? Find the hidden message in the remaining letters:**

T	C	H	E	S	T	H	A	I	R	K	E	E	P	S
M	R	E	E	P	U	L	S	E	R	A	T	E	Y	N
H	A	E	L	A	P	A	I	N	L	E	S	S	O	O
T	H	T	A	E	R	B	F	O	T	R	O	H	S	I
Y	N	B	A	T	C	T	C	O	N	N	E	C	T	T
H	O	L	E	D	M	T	B	A	E	V	A	H	S	A
R	I	A	W	R	L	E	R	E	N	W	R	I	S	T
T	T	N	U	A	U	A	N	O	A	K	R	H	E	I
R	A	K	A	R	T	S	N	T	D	T	L	T	H	P
A	C	E	E	A	L	C	A	O	T	E	T	E	H	L
E	I	T	W	I	R	E	H	E	S	A	S	Y	X	A
H	D	E	L	C	Y	C	I	B	M	R	B	A	J	P
H	E	A	R	T	A	T	T	A	C	K	E	L	Z	H
I	M	N	I	A	P	T	S	E	H	C	C	P	E	B
B	L	O	O	D	P	R	E	S	S	U	R	E	Q	C

....

....

....

....

....

....

....

....

Hidden message: ....

8 Spirometry

LISTENING Track 9

1 **Listen to the dialog and answer the following questions:**

- *What examination is being performed?*
- *What does the medical assistant do?*

READING

2 **Read the text and check new words in the vocabulary list or in a dictionary:**

pulmonary, spirometry, spirometer, obstructive diseases, tissue, fibrosis, restrictive diseases, cough, asthma, lung emphysema, bronchitis, bronchodilator inhaler, reversibility testing, microorganism, maneuver, expiratory

A pulmonary[1] function test (called "spirometry") measures the volume of air that you can blow out of the lungs. A spirometer has a mouthpiece that the patient uses to blow into the device[2]. Some conditions mean that a person cannot inhale a normal volume of air. Causes may be the narrowing of airways (obstructive diseases) or conditions that damage the lung tissue[3] itself such as scarring[4] or fibrosis[5] of the lung (restrictive[6] diseases).

Indications for a pulmonary function test:

- coughing
- breathing problems
- lung diseases (e.g. asthma, COPD[7], lung emphysema, bronchitis)
- before operations
- therapy control

How to prepare for the test:

Do not eat a heavy meal, do not smoke for 24 hours, do not drink alcohol and do not exercise up to a few hours before the test. Specific instructions may include not to use bronchodilator[8] inhalers before the test.

In reversibility testing[9], medication may be inhaled before the test. This test is to see if your airways open wider with medication or not.

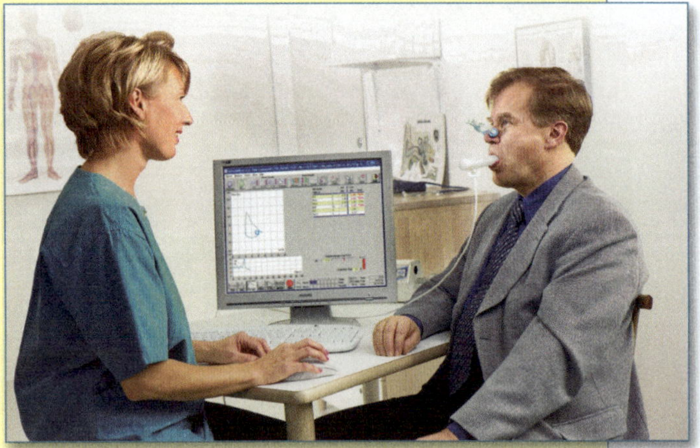

Procedure:

During the test, a clip is put onto the patient's nose so that no air can escape through the nose. After breathing in fully, the patient is asked to close his/her lips around the mouthpiece of the spirometer.

Breathing maneuvers:

At first the patient has to breathe in and out normally and evenly, continuing until there is a cracking noise. Then, the patient is asked to take the deepest breath possible, and then exhale into the sensor as far and long as possible.

In a further maneuver[10] the patient has to breathe in fully and then blow out as forcefully[11] and far as possible. This is directly followed by a rapid[12] inhalation (inspiration).

1 pulmonary – relating to the lungs, medical term
2 device – Gerät
3 tissue – Gewebe
4 scarring – Vernarbung
5 fibrosis – Fibrose (krankhafte Vermehrung des Bindegewebes)
6 restrictive – restriktiv (einschränkend, begrenzend)
7 COPD = chronic obstructive lung disease
8 bronchodilator – medication to widen the bronchi
9 reversibility testing – Bronchospasmolysetest
10 maneuver – Manöver
11 forcefully – strongly, with power
12 rapid – quick

Generally, the medical assistant will give the patient instructions about what to do and allow the patient to practice what is expected[13] of him. This motivates the patient to do the best he or she can do and achieve[14] a better test result.

Risks:
The risk is minimal for most people, although there is a slight risk of a collapsed lung in some patients with lung or heart disease.

Results:
Normal results are based on a person's age, height, weight and sex. The measured results are expressed[15] in percentage of the normal results.
The most common measurements used are:
FEV1 – Forced Expiratory Volume in one second. This is the amount[16] of air you can exhale in one second.
FVC – Forced Vital Capacity. This is the total amount of air that you can breathe out in one breath.

13 expected – erwartet
14 to achieve – erreichen
15 expressed – ausgedrückt
16 amount – Menge

COMPREHENSION

3 **Answer the questions below:**

1. What can you measure with spirometry?

   ....

2. When is this test performed?

   ....

   ....

3. Name the "don't s" the patient has to follow before the test.

   ....

   ....

4. How do you avoid that air escapes through the patient's nose?

   ....

5. What does the patient have to do with the mouthpiece?

   ....

6. Which instruction do you have to give for the first breathing maneuver? Write it down as if you were giving instructions to the patient.

   ....

7. What instructions do you have to give when measuring dynamic volumes (e.g. FVC)? Write it down as if you were giving instructions to the patient.

   ....

8. What does the medical assistant have to do to get the best results from the patient?

   ....

   ....

9. What are the results dependent on?

   ....

4 **True or false? Correct false sentences:**

	T/F
1. An indication for a pulmonary function test is nose bleeding.	
2. You should not eat a heavy meal before the test.	
3. The test is performed to measure how much oxygen you have in your blood.	
4. Only the doctor is allowed to perform the pulmonary function test because there is a high risk of a lung collapse.	
5. In some cases you have to perform a pulmonary function test before the patient has an operation.	
6. Before the examination you have to write down the patient's age, height, weight, sex and if he/she has any allergies.	
7. It is possible that the patient feels dizzy during the test.	
8. The patient has to bring his/her own nose clip.	
9. If a patient is already taking medication you do not have to perform a pulmonary function test.	

DIALOG / ROLEPLAY

5 **Work with a partner. Write a dialog between Ms. Andersson (patient) and the MA:**

Der MFA begrüßt die Patientin.

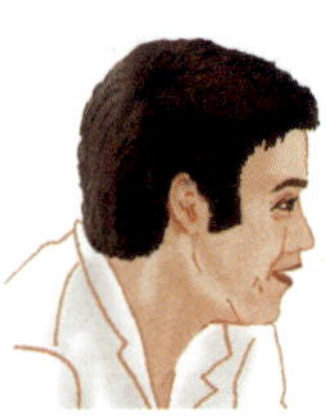

....

Patientin stellt sich vor, gibt an, dass sie einen Termin zum Lungenfunktionstest hat.

....

....

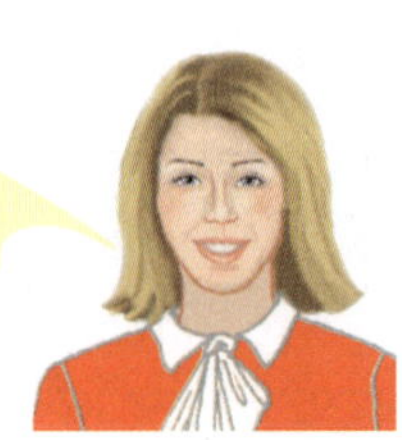

Der MFA führt die Patientin zum Behandlungsraum...
Er bittet die Patientin Platz zu nehmen, informiert sie, dass ein Lungenfunktionstest zur Messung des Lungenvolumens durchgeführt wird. Dazu benötigt und erfragt er die Daten der Patientin.

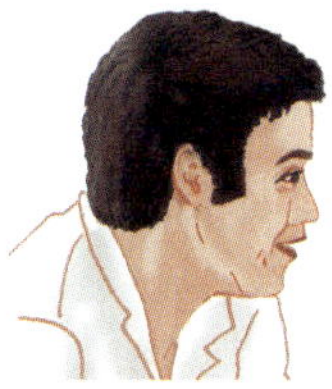

Patientin antwortet.

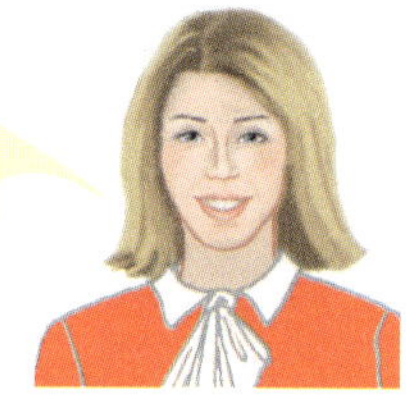

Der MFA fragt, ob die Patientin raucht, Bronchienerweiterungsmittel genommen hat und ob sie eine Zahnprothese trägt.

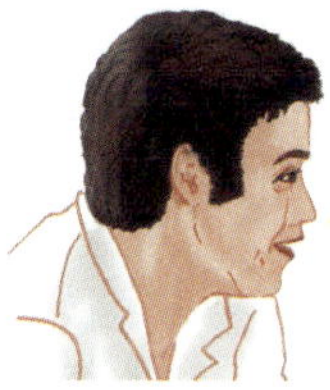

Patientin antwortet.

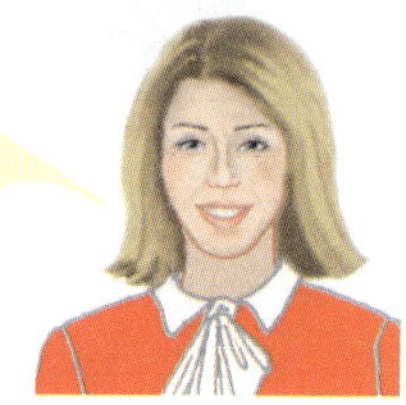

Der MFA erklärt, dass die Patientin eine Nasenklammer bekommt, damit keine Luft durch die Nase entweichen kann.

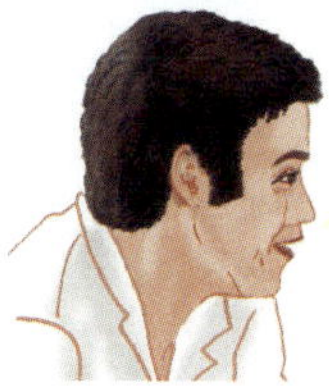

Patientin fragt, ob das weh tut.

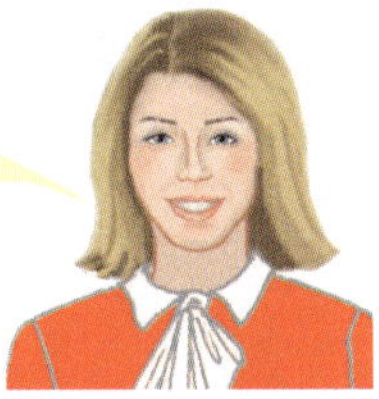

Der MFA erklärt, dass das etwas unangenehm aber notwendig ist. Er setzt ein neues Mundstück auf das Gerät...
Die Patientin soll jetzt aufstehen und die Nasenklammer aufsetzen. Der MFA erklärt das erste Atemkommando und führt es dann mit der Patientin durch:
Die Patientin soll normal ein- und ausatmen, dann so tief wie möglich einatmen und alles wieder vollständig ausatmen:

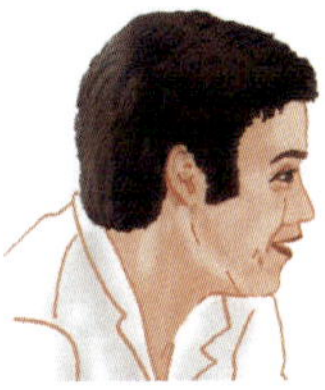

Der MFA erklärt das zweite Atemmanöver.
Dabei soll die Patientin, wie zuvor, erst normal ein- und ausatmen und dann, wie zuvor, so tief wie möglich einatmen.
Anschließend muss die Patientin die gesamte Luft so schnell und kraftvoll wie möglich mit Schwung ausatmen. Der MFA demonstriert der Patientin, wie sie zu atmen hat.
Anschließend lobt er die Patientin und fragt, wie es ihr geht.

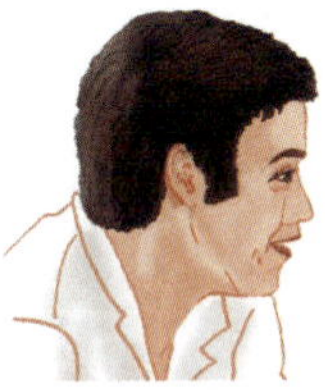

Der Patientin ist etwas schwindelig, sonst ist alles o.k., sie bedankt sich.

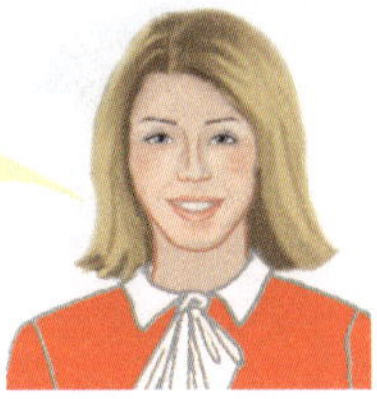

Der MFA teilt der Patientin mit, dass sie die Nasenklammer jetzt abnehmen und sich setzen darf, bietet ihr etwas Wasser zu trinken an und teilt ihr mit, dass die Ärztin gleich die Ergebnisse mit ihr besprechen wird.

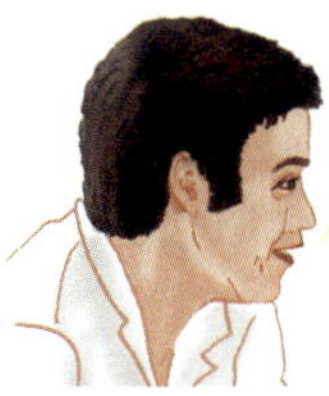

....

....

....

....

Spirometry WORD SEARCH

6 **Can you find 21 English words in the puzzle? Write them down and translate them into German:**

R	F	V	E	I	D	Y	X	B	E	C	E	L	G	W
T	O	Q	M	L	X	F	R	F	S	V	A	R	F	G
H	R	T	I	O	E	U	S	S	I	T	G	N	U	L
G	C	A	A	U	U	C	T	T	O	R	C	F	V	K
I	E	M	H	L	O	T	C	H	N	I	M	N	Y	C
E	F	O	F	P	I	U	H	E	G	A	L	Q	R	O
W	U	U	D	D	R	D	L	P	N	I	E	G	A	U
P	L	N	L	T	E	A	O	I	I	M	E	U	N	G
Y	L	T	S	A	H	N	E	H	K	E	T	H	O	H
J	Y	B	A	N	M	B	T	V	C	S	C	Q	M	I
H	O	M	I	B	Z	X	G	U	A	N	R	E	L	N
O	S	P	I	R	O	M	E	T	R	Y	O	K	U	G
S	Y	A	W	R	I	A	P	S	C	E	F	R	P	L
E	X	H	A	L	E	K	S	U	F	Y	S	T	B	U
E	J	N	O	S	E	C	L	I	P	X	J	N	I	C

....

....

....

....

....

....

....

....

....

....

....

....

....

....

....

....

....

....

....

....

....

German translation:

....

....

....

....

....

....

9 Arterial Blood Gas Analysis

LISTENING Track 10

1 **Listen to the dialog and answer the following questions:**

- *What examination is being performed?*
- *Try to describe the procedure.*

READING

2 **Read the following text and find the German words 3. Check any other new vocabulary in the vocabulary list or in a dictionary.**

analysis, oxygen, carbon dioxide, acidity, respiratory, hyperventilation, bicarbonate, anemia, artery, capillary, diagnosis

Blood gas analysis, also called arterial blood gas (ABG) analysis, is a test that measures how much oxygen and carbon dioxide are in your arterial blood. Oxygen in the lungs is carried to the red blood cells and from there to the tissues[1] through the body. It also checks the acidity[2] (pH) of your blood and therefore gives information about the body's acid-base balance[3].

Why is the test performed ?

The test may indicate a respiratory (lung/breathing), metabolic[4], or kidney disorder. Symptoms include difficulty breathing, shortness of breath, or rapid breathing (hyperventilation). It helps determine the effectiveness of oxygen therapy.

Normal blood gas values[5] are as follows:

Partial pressure of oxygen[6] (PaO_2): 75–100 mm Hg
Partial pressure of carbon dioxide[7] ($PaCO_2$): 35–45 mm Hg
Oxygen content[8] (O_2CT): 15–23%
Oxygen saturation[9] (SaO_2): 94–100%
Bicarbonate (HCO_3): 22–26 mEq/liter
PH: 7.35–7.45.

Values that differ from those listed above may indicate respiratory, metabolic, or kidney disease. Disorders such as anemia can produce an abnormally low oxygen value.

Capillary blood test

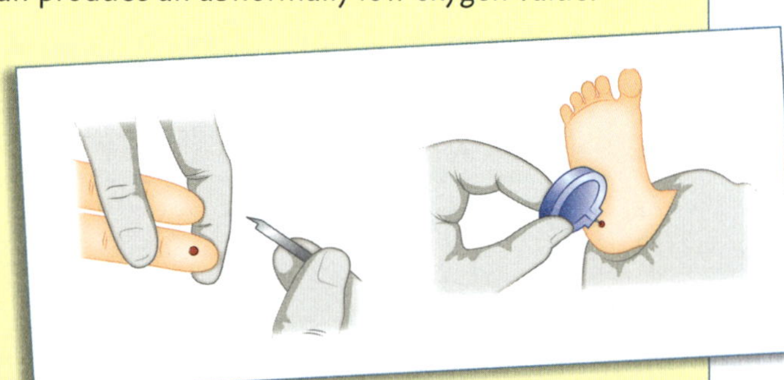

Blood gas analysis is performed on blood from an artery or capillary. Capillary blood tests are often performed in the doctor's practice when only a small amount of blood is needed. Because patients are often afraid of skin punctures, it is important to reassure them. Before you start, let the patient know what you are going to do to get their cooperation. You should tell the patient that there will be a little pain during the skin puncture, but that it will not last long. Tell the patient that this is necessary for the doctor to make a diagnosis. When procedures are done correctly, the patient should feel minimal discomfort. The most practical sites to use are the ring finger, the earlobe and in infants the heel. Before the puncture an ointment that increases[10] the local blood flow is sometimes used.

1 tissue – Gewebe
2 acidity – Säuregehalt
3 acid-base balance – Säure-Base-Hauhalt
4 metabolic – auf den Stoffwechsel bezogen
5 value – Wert
6 partial pressure of oxygen – Sauerstoffpartialdruck
7 partial pressure of carbon dioxide – Kohlendioxidpartialdruck
8 oxygen content – Sauerstoffgehalt
9 oxygen saturation – Sauerstoffsättigung
10 to increase – erhöhen

COMPREHENSION

3 **Find the following words in the text:**

Blutgasanalyse – Sauerstoff – Kohlenstoffdioxid – Körpergewebe
Rote Blutkörperchen – Säure-Basen-Haushalt – Kurzatmigkeit
Wirkung – Stoffwechselkrankheit – Erkrankung des Atmungssystems
Blutarmut – geringe Menge – Arterie – Stelle – beruhigen
Mitarbeit – Unbehagen – dauern

4 **Match the materials you need with the correct picture:**

gloves – disinfectant – swabs – lancet – ointment – capillary tube

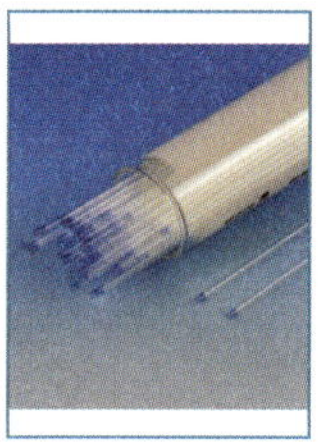

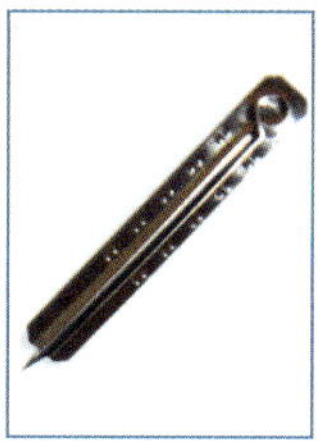

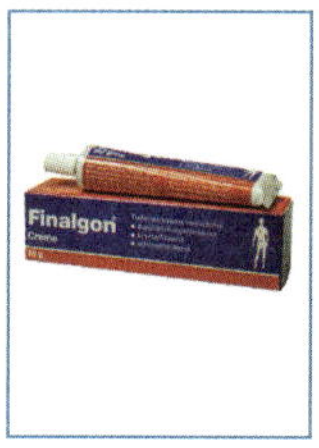

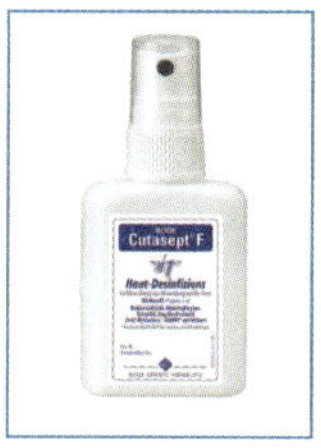

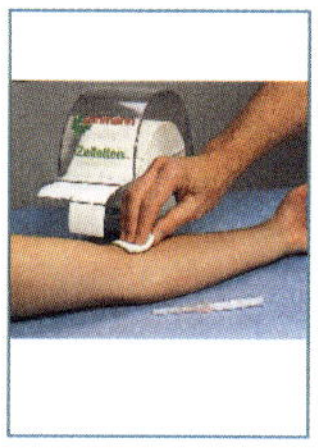

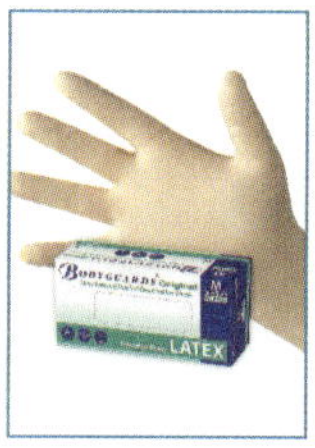

....

You have to prick the earlobe very fast without hesitating. Don't press the earlobe too hard because this can lead to an inaccurate result. Make sure that there are no gas bubbles in the blood sample.

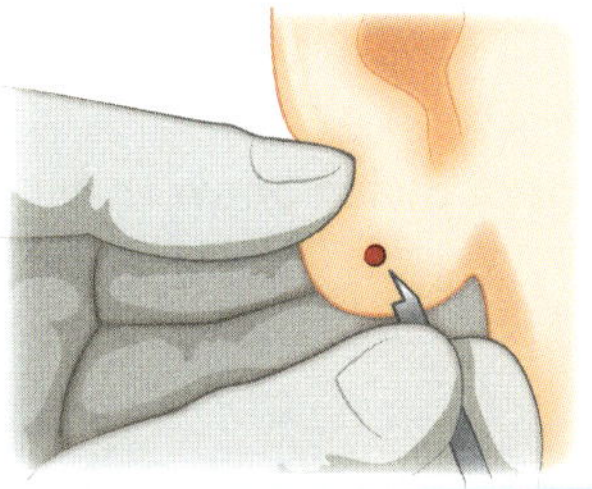

Arterial Blood Gas CRISS CROSS

5 **Fill in the crossword Puzzle:**

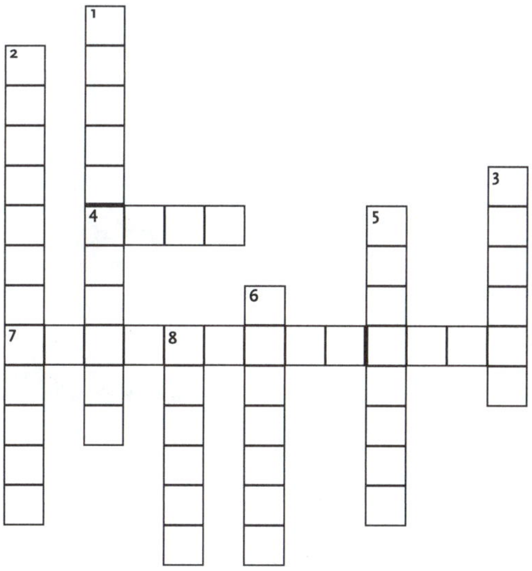

Across

4. piece of absorbent material for medical use
7. you use this to take the blood from the earlobe

Down

1. small amount of red body fluid you use for blood tests
2. a fluid you use to avoid infection
3. you put them on your hands to protect yourself from disease
5. a creamy substance that you can apply on your skin
6. the most frequently pierced body part
8. a small needle to prick the skin

COMPREHENSION

6 **Answer the following questions:**

1. What does the abbreviation ABG stand for?
2. What does the test measure?
3. What kind of disorders can be diagnosed?
4. What kind of blood do you need to perform the test?
5. How much blood do you need?
6. Which puncture sites can be used?
7. What can you do to make the patient feel more at ease?

DIALOG / ROLEPLAY

Work with a partner. Write a dialog between Mr. Ninh (patient) and you (MA). Fill in the empty bubbles:

MFA begrüßt Patient.

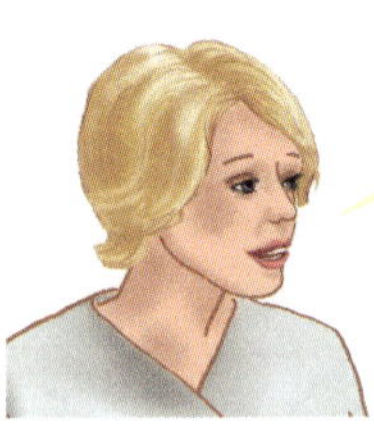

Patient stellt sich vor, er hat einen Termin zur Blutgasanalyse (BGA).

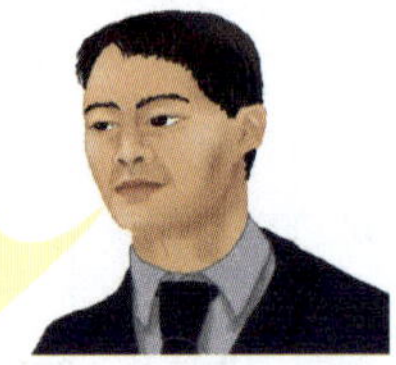

MFA sagt dem Patienten, dass er sich in den Behandlungsraum setzen soll, welcher sich am Ende des Ganges rechts befindet.

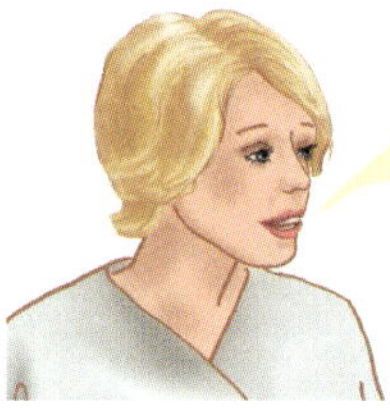

Patient ist ängstlich und fragt, ob es weh tun wird.

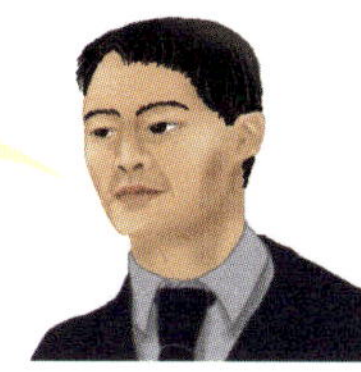

MFA beruhigt den Patienten.

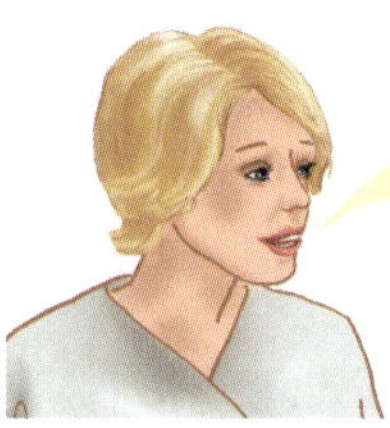

Patient fragt, warum die Untersuchung durchgeführt wird.

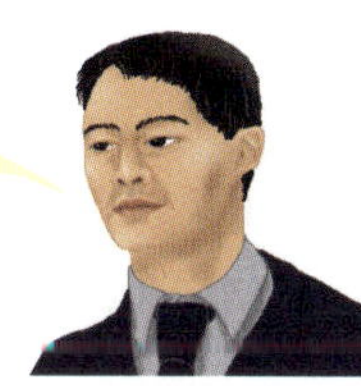

MFA erklärt, dass die Messung durchgeführt wird, um den Sauerstoff- und CO_2-Wert im Blut zu ermitteln. Der Arzt benötigt diese Werte, um die Lunge des Patienten zu überprüfen.

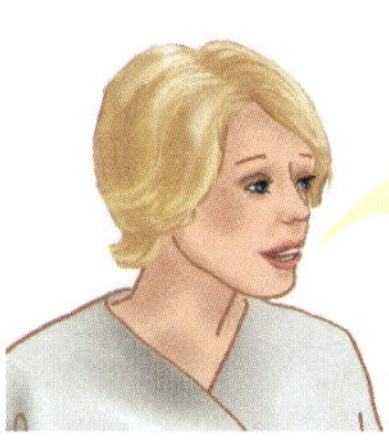

Patient fragt, was die MFA jetzt tun wird.

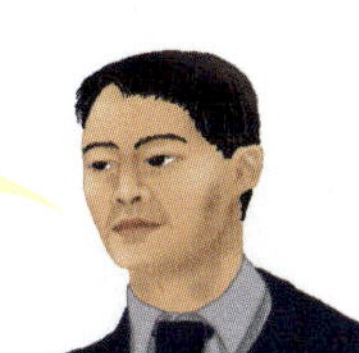

MFA erklärt dem Patienten die Untersuchung: Zuerst wird eine durchblutungsfördernde Salbe auf das Ohrläppchen aufgetragen, die kurz einwirken muss. Dann wird die Stelle mit einem Alkoholtupfer desinfiziert. Es wird mit einer kleinen Lanzette gestochen und eine Blutprobe entnommen. Dies kann ein wenig weh tun.
Zum Schluss versorgt sie den Patienten mit einem Pflaster.

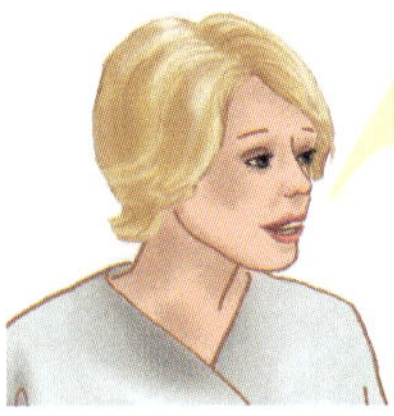

Patient sagt, dass er kaum etwas gemerkt hat.

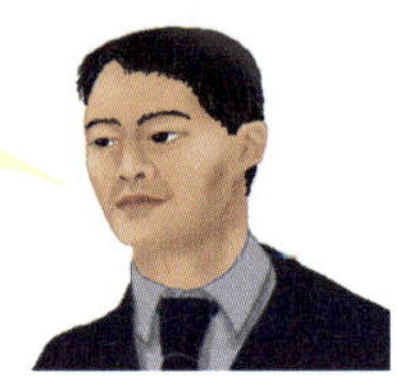

MFA bittet den Patienten, im Wartezimmer Platz zu nehmen.

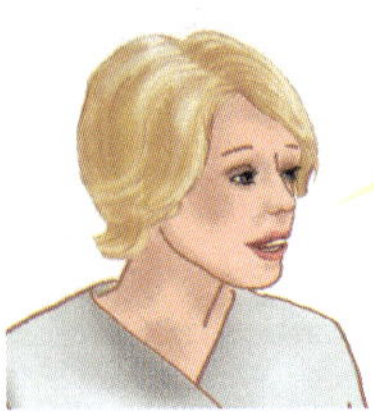

10 Urinary Tract Infections

READING

1 **Read the following information and check the words in bold print in the vocabulary list or in a dictionary:**

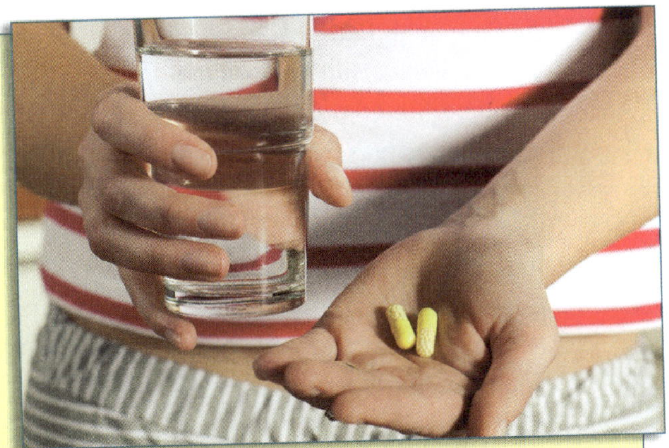

What is the urinary tract?
The urinary tract produces and stores urine, one of your body's waste products[1]. The urine travels from the ***kidneys*** down two narrow[2] tubes, the ***ureters***. It is then stored in the ***bladder***. When the bladder is about half full, you may begin to feel the need to empty it by ***urinating***. Normal urine contains no ***bacteria***. Bacteria (or "***germs***") may, at times, get into the urinary tract (and the urine). A urinary tract infection (***UTI***) is an infection of the bladder (***cystitis***) and sometimes the kidneys can also be involved (***pyelonephritis***). It is important to treat UTIs so that the kidneys are not damaged. Most uncomplicated UTIs occur[3] in otherwise ***healthy*** and sexually active women. Contamination of the urinary tract occurs more often in women than in men because the female ***urethra*** (the tube that goes from the bladder out of the body) is shorter and closer to the sources[4] of bacteria, the ***anus*** and the ***vagina***.

What are the signs of a urinary tract infection?
Your need to urinate may seem ***urgent*** and ***frequent***; but when you try to do so you may only produce a few drops of urine. You may feel a ***painful burning sensation*** as the urine comes out. You may notice that the urine has an ***unpleasant smell*** or a ***cloudy look***. At times, bladder infections may also cause lower back pain, fever, or ***chills***.

How do you find out whether you have a UTI?
You can only find out whether you have a urinary tract infection by consulting a doctor. The doctor can diagnose an infection through a simple ***urine test***, which detects[5] the presence of ***white blood cells*** and bacteria in the urine.

How are these infections treated?
Urinary tract infections are treated with oral antibiotics (infection-fighting drugs). Your doctor will choose a drug that treats the infection and you will get ***dosage instructions***. Take the antibiotic exactly as told by the doctor. Take the medicine until all the pills are gone – even if symptoms disappear – to make sure that all of the bacteria have been killed. Once the laboratory test results are in, the doctor may switch to another antibiotic, one that is more effective against the bacteria found in your urine.
Before antibiotics begin ***to take effect***, some ***discomfort*** can be ***eased*** with a ***heating pad*** and ***painkillers*** like paracetamol or ibuprofen.
Drink plenty of water or ***herbal tea*** to ***flush*** bacteria from the urinary tract. Drinking ***cranberry juice*** may stop bacteria from sticking to the bladder wall.
Don't have sex until your cystitis has been cured.

urinary tract, urine, ureters, cystitis, pyelonephritis, urethra, vagina, dosage, laboratory, bowel movement, menstruation

1 waste products – Abfallprodukte
2 narrow – eng
3 to occur – auftreten, vorkommen
4 source – Quelle
5 to detect – ausfindig machen, aufspüren

What steps can you take to help prevent these infections?

You can take the following steps to reduce your risk of getting a urinary tract infection:

- Always empty your bladder when you feel the ***urge*** – don't wait.
- Wash the ***genital area*** with water, not soap.
- Wipe yourself correctly from front to back, especially after a ***bowel movement***, to avoid the ***spread*** of bacteria from the ***rectum*** to the urethra.
- Drink enough ***fluids*** each day, especially water.
- Wear loose[6] ***cotton underpants***.
- Avoid perfumed products. The use of bubble bath or perfumed soaps in the vaginal area may increase[7] the risk of UTIs.
- Tampons and ***sanitary napkins*** should be changed frequently during menstruation.
- Practice safe sexual habits. A woman's risk of developing a UTI may be lowered by washing the external genital area before ***sexual intercourse***, and urinating after sexual intercourse to get rid of[8] any germs.
- Live a healthy lifestyle. Stress, ***fatigue*** and a poor diet[9] can all affect the immune system, increasing the risk of infection.
- Consult your doctor at the first sign of a problem. Urinary tract infections are very common[10], and they are easier to treat if caught before they become severe[11].

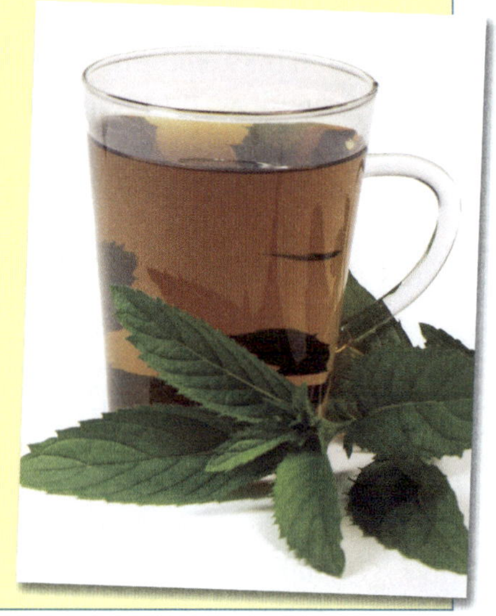

6 loose – locker
7 to increase – erhöhen
8 to get rid of – loswerden
9 diet – Ernährung
10 to be common – hier: weit verbreitet, häufig
11 severe – schwerwiegend, ernst

COMPREHENSION

2 **Fill in the gaps with the following words from the text above:**

antibiotics, anus, bowel movement, bladder, burning sensation, chills, cloudy, cotton, cystitis, discomfort, dosage instructions, frequent, germs, herbal tea, immune system, kidney, sanitary napkins, sexual intercourse, smell, urge, urgent, ureter, urethra (2x), urinary tract infection, urinate, urine, vagina, waste products, white blood cells

1. .... and .... are all organs of the urinary tract.
2. The function of the kidneys is to clean the blood of .... by producing ....
3. Another word for passing urine is to ....
4. Another word for bacteria or micro organisms is .... They may cause UTI (..). The medical term for bladder infection is ....

5. Sources of bacteria are the .... and ....
6. Because the female .... is shorter than the male version, women get cystitis more easily.
7. Symptoms of cystitis are .... and .... urination, a .... during urination and sometimes ....
8. The urine looks .... and often has a foul ....
9. A urine test mostly shows bacteria and ....
10. UTIs are treated with .... which are prescribed by a doctor. Drinking plenty of water or .... also eases discomfort.
11. It is very important to stick to the .... to make sure that all the bacteria have been killed.
12. Don't have .... while suffering from cystitis.
13. To avoid bladder infection, wear .... underpants, wipe correctly after .... and change tampons or .... frequently. Don't wait to go to the toilet if you feel the .... to urinate.
14. To strengthen your .... you should eat healthy food and avoid stress.

3 **In which sentences can you find the following information about cystitis? Match the numbers from the sentences above to the letters below.**

a) definition
b) causes
c) symptoms
d) diagnosis
e) treatment
f) prevention

DIALOG / ROLEPLAY

4 **Working with a partner, write a dialog between you and your friend. Include information on topics a) to f). Be prepared to present it in class.**

Your best friend met a new boyfriend last month. Now she is showing symptoms of bladder infection and is really worried. She knows that you are training to be a medical assistant so asks you for advice.

11 Midstream Specimen of Urine (MSU)

LISTENING Track 11

1 **Listen to the dialog and answer the following questions:**

- *What examination is being performed?*
- *What instructions does the medical assistant give?*

READING

2 **Read the following text and check any new vocabulary in the word list or in a dictionary:**

Midstream Specimen of Urine, urine, leucocytes, antibiotics, cystitis, sterile, urethra, vagina, menstruation

1 MSU – Mittelstrahlurin
2 UTI (Urinary Tract Infection) – Harnwegsinfekt
3 various – verschieden
4 suspect – Verdacht
5 aim – Ziel
6 germs – Keime
7 urethra – Urethra/Harnröhre
8 cleansing wipes – Reinigungstücher
9 labia – Schamlippen
10 disposable – Einweg
11 provided – bereitgestellt
12 traces – Spuren
13 detergent – Reinigungsmittel

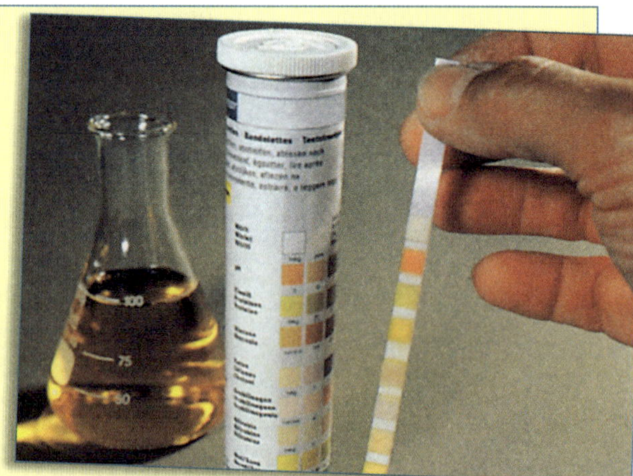

Why MSU?

The Midstream Specimen of Urine (MSU)[1] is tested to look for urinary tract infections (UTI)[2]. Typical symptoms of a UTI are a burning pain when you pass urine and the need to pass urine very often.

The urine sample contains bacteria and white blood cells (leucocytes) and sometimes also blood or protein. If the bacteria travels further up, the kidneys could become infected. If the urine tests positive for bacteria, the bacteria is then tested against various[3] antibiotics. Finally, the doctor can prescribe the most effective antibiotic. During treatment the patient should drink a lot of water to help flush the bacteria out of the bladder.

If cystitis (bladder inflammation) is suspected[4] the urine test is a quick examination. The aim[5] is to get a urine sample from the middle of the bladder. Normally, this urine is sterile. The first bit of urine that you pass may have been contaminated with germs[6] from the urethra[7].

Collection of MSU

The patient has to wash her/his hands and genital area before collecting a urine sample. In the doctor's practice this can be done with moist cleansing wipes[8]. Women have to hold open the labia[9] – the entrance of the vagina. Men have to pull back the foreskin. Then the first urine flows into the toilet to wash germs out of the urethra. Without stopping the flow of urine, the patient then has to catch some urine in a disposable[10] cup which is usually provided[11] by the doctor. After enough urine has been collected the rest of the urine can be passed into the toilet.

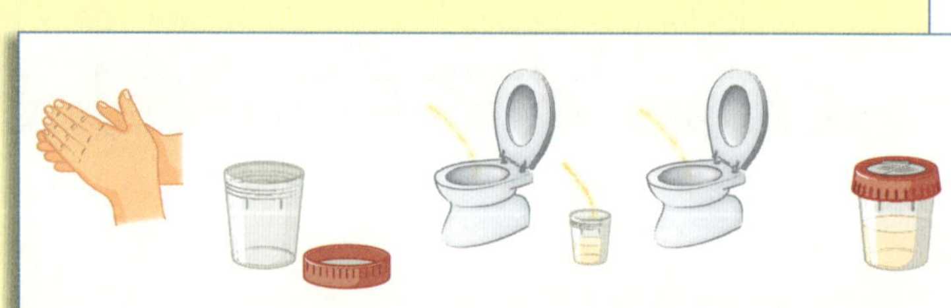

For optimal results the patient has to bring the urine sample back to the doctor's practice within two hours. If this is not possible, the sample can be kept in the fridge for a maximum of two hours.

It is not possible to do the test during menstruation because the menstruation could falsify the result. Jam jars should not be used for the sample as they may contain traces[12] of sugar or detergent[13] that could falsify the result.

COMPREHENSION

3 **Match the words with their definitions:**

1. MSU	a. infection fighting drug
2. UTI	b. white blood cells
3. urethra	c. bladder inflammation
4. germs	d. urinary tract infection
5. disposable	e. to clean the inside of the body by using a lot of liquid
6. detergent	f. free from micro organisms
7. frequently	g. change something to be untrue
8. leucocytes	h. midstream specimen of urine
9. antibiotic	i. skin covering the end of the penis
10. sterile	j. very small organisms/micro organisms
11. cystitis	k. product is designed to be thrown away after it has been used
12. to flush	l. powder or liquid for washing things
13. labia	m. often
14. foreskin	n. tube leading from the bladder outside of the body
15. (re)fridge(rator)	o. entrance to the vagina
16. to falsify	p. big cupboard which keeps food cool

4 **Answer the following questions:**

1. When do you need MSU?

   ....

2. Why is it important to catch a urine sample from the middle of the bladder?

   ....

3. Is it possible to do the (midstream) urine test during menstruation? Why or why not?

   ....

4. When should you bring the urine sample back to the doctor's office?

   ....

5. Does it matter what kind of container is used for the sample? Explain.

   ....

   ....

6. How is cystitis treated?

   ....

DIALOG / ROLEPLAY

5 **Write a dialog with a partner. Complete the speech bubbles:**

Mr. Benton has been suffering from terrible pain in his bladder for the last five hours. That's why he decides to consult his GP. Now he is at the doctor's practice.

MFA begrüßt den Patienten.

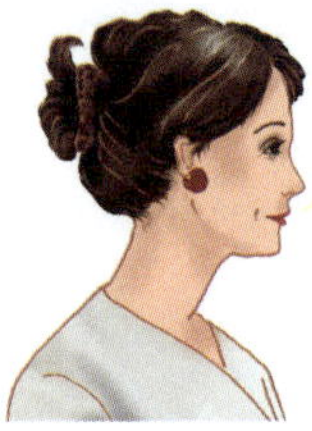

....

Patient möchte den Arzt sehen, da er fürchterliche Schmerzen beim Wasserlassen hat. Er hat keinen Termin.

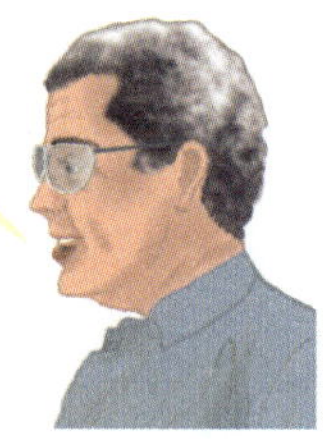

....

....

....

MFA fragt, um was für einen Schmerz es sich handelt.

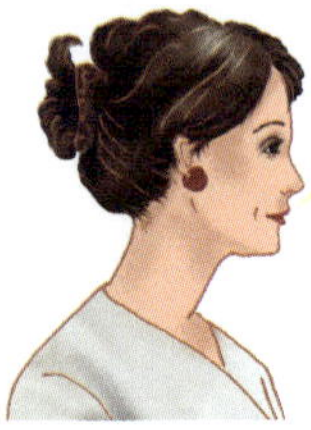

....

....

Patient sagt, dass es sich um einen brennenden Schmerz in der Blase handelt und er ständigen Harndrang hat.

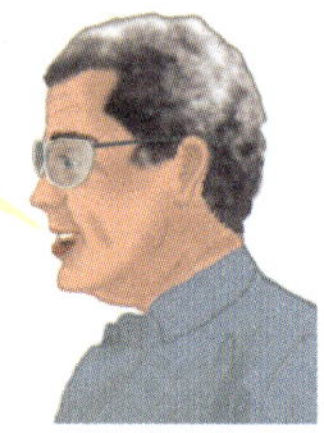

....

....

MFA sagt, dass es sich nach einer Blasenentzündung anhört. Der Patient soll auf die Toilette gehen, wo er auch die Urinbecher findet. Sie sagt ihm, wo sich die Toilette befindet, bittet den Patienten um Gewinnung von Mittelstrahlurin und fragt ihn, ob er weiß, wie man diesen gewinnt.

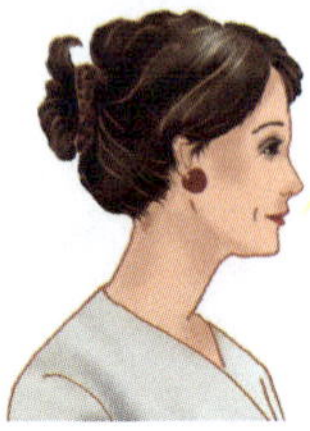

....

....

....

....

Patient verneint dieses und fragt, wie er vorgehen soll.

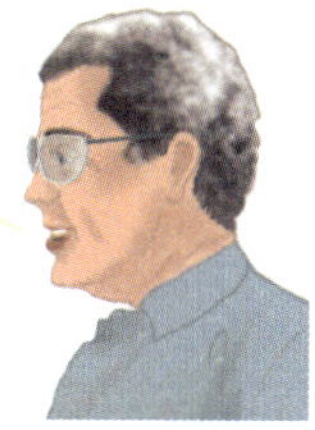

MFA bittet um Säuberung der Hände und des Genitalbereichs mit den bereitgestellten Tupfern. Sie erklärt ihm, wie er den Mittelstrahlurin gewinnt. Anschließend soll er den Urin in das Fenster stellen und noch im Wartezimmer Platz nehmen, bis er aufgerufen wird.

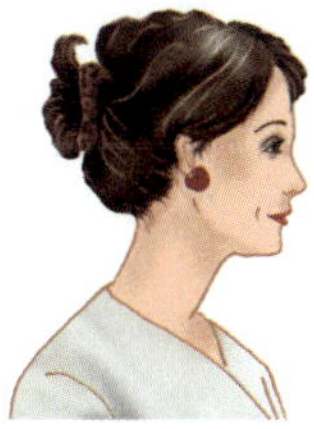

6 **With a partner write a dialog giving Ms. Mason instructions on how to collect an MSU at home.**

Ms. Mason shows symptoms of a UTI when she arrives at her GP. She has been going to the toilet all morning and is not able to pass any more urine because her bladder is completely empty. You ask her to collect an MSU at home the next morning.

MSU WORD SEARCH

7 **Can you find 18 hidden words? Find the hidden message in the remaining letters:**

```
N B A C T E R I A S D E P
R O U R I C D N I K N L R
A P I L E O E T O I T P E
S O F T O S I L A W P M S
L A R L A T U P L H T A C
A E B E S M G L A O E S R
T R G Y D N M R T F C E I
I P C D I D M A L F V N P
N R J N I A A U L J E I T
E P R C C R S L A F S R I
G U L Y J H F E B B N U O
B A N T I B I O T I C I N
S M R E G F O R E S K I N
```

Hidden message: ....

12 Taking Antibiotics

LISTENING Track 12

1 **Listen to the dialog and answer the following questions:**

- *What medicine is prescribed?*
- *How does the patient have to take the drug?*

READING

2 **Read the following text and check any new words in the vocabulary list or in the dictionary:**

antibiotic, tonsillitis, urinary, respiratory, penicillin, pregnancy, contraception, pharmacist,

1 range – Bandbreite
2 previous – vorhergehende
3 with caution – mit Vorsicht
4 to interact – wechselwirken
5 dairy products – Milchprodukte
6 to interfere – hier: behindern
7 absorption – Absorption, Aufnahme
8 patient information leaflet – Packungsbeilage
9 to apply – hier: gelten

Antibiotics are medicines that kill bacteria which cause infection. They are used to treat a wide range[1] of infections, e.g. tonsillitis, urinary and respiratory tract infections, scarlet fever. There are many different types of antibiotics. The type of antibiotic you take will depend on the type of infection you have. Antibiotics destroy the cell walls of bacteria so that the bacteria die. You should complete your course of antibiotics as instructed by your doctor, even if you feel better. If you stop taking antibiotics too early, it can lead to the bacteria becoming resistant to antibiotics. This makes them harder to kill.

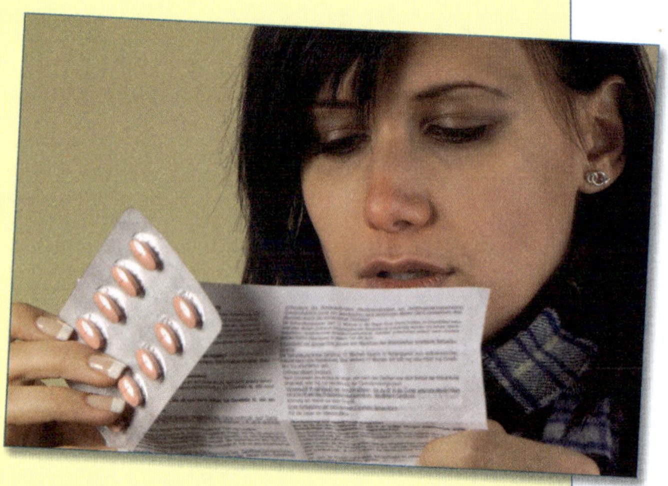

Special considerations

You should avoid taking penicillin if you have had a previous[2] allergic reaction to penicillin. You should take antibiotics with caution[3] if you have kidney and liver problems. If you are pregnant or breastfeeding, most antibiotics should only be used when absolutely necessary. Tell your physician if you are pregnant or breastfeeding, so that they can prescribe the most suitable antibiotic for you.

Interactions and Side effects

Antibiotics can sometimes interact[4] with other medicines, e.g. antibiotics may cause your contraceptive pill to become less effective at preventing pregnancy. Women taking the contraceptive pill should use an additional method of contraception (for example, condoms) while taking antibiotics.
There are some antibiotics where you should not drink milk or eat dairy products[5] at the same time as taking the antibiotic. This is because the calcium in the dairy product interferes[6] with the absorption[7] of the antibiotic, so it is less effective.
If you want to check for more drug interactions ask your doctor or local pharmacist or read the patient information leaflet[8] that comes with your medication. The same applies[9] for side effects.
Take antibiotics as written on the packet or patient information leaflet, or as you've been told by your GP or pharmacist.

Remember: To avoid bacteria becoming resistant to an antibiotic, you have to complete your course of antibiotics as directed by your doctor, even if you feel better.

COMPREHENSION

3 Match the words with their definitions:

1. tonsillitis	a. can not be harmed
2. respiratory tract	b. a medicine a woman uses to prevent pregnancy
3. resistant	c. you get ill or get a rash from a normally harmless substance
4. physician	d. another word for medication
5. contraceptive pill	e. breathing organs
6. pharmacist	f. an infection-fighting drug
7. antibiotic	g. infection of the throat
8. allergic reaction	h. milk and food made from milk
9. dairy product	i. doctor
10. drug	j. a person who prepares and sells medicines

4 Are the following statements true (T) or false (F)? Correct false statements.

	T/F
1. Antibiotics are drugs that fight viral infections.	
2. Penicillin is one type of antibiotic.	
3. The type of antibiotic you take is independent of the kind of infection you have.	
4. As soon as you feel better you can stop taking antibiotics.	
5. Bacteria may become resistant to an antibiotic.	
6. Many people show allergic reactions to penicillin.	
7. Everybody can take antibiotics.	
8. There are no interactions with the contraceptive pill.	
9. You should be careful with contraception while taking antibiotics.	
10. The only way to know about side effects is to ask your doctor.	
11. Many antibiotics mustn't be taken with milk.	

DOSAGE INSTRUCTIONS

Mrs. Mason has been diagnosed with cystitis. The doctor has prescribed Ciprobay Uro® Filmtabletten. You have printed out the prescription and hand it over to her. Now she wants to know how she has to take the tablets. You have a look at the "Rote Liste".

5 **Write her a short note. Use the two squares below as a help.**

Dosage instruction

Ciprobay Uro® Filmtabletten

Dos. 2mal tgl.1 Filmtabl. Bei unkomplizierten Infektionen der ableitenden Harnwege der Frau kann eine 3-tägige Behandlungsdauer ausreichen.

Taking medicine / Dosage instructions

Take	one two three etc.	tablet(s)/ capsule(s), drops/ globules	with (a lot of) water on an empty stomach	before/with/ after meals (breakfast/dinner) in the morning/evening
Don't chew				
You mustn't take more than				a day/within 24 hours.
Swallow Drink	the	medicine		before you go to bed.
Dissolve		effervescent tablet(s)	in water	
Apply		ointment/lotion/ creme/gel	thinly/thickly	once/twice/ three times a day.
Insert		suppository	into the anus/ vagina	
Inject		insulin	into the abdomen/ into the thigh	

Possible side effects:
The medicine may cause...
...nausea, headache, drowsiness stomach upset, diarrhea, dizziness, redness, swelling, pain, etc.

Note:
You can buy medicine in a pharmacy
– on prescription
– over the counter

You take a medicine ***for*** a symptom/illness/disease.

6 **Translate the dosage instructions below. What is the medicine for? Use the "Rote Liste".**

Buscopan® plus	Erw. 1-2 Filmtbl. 3mal tgl. unzerkaut mit Flüssigkeit od. 1 Zäpfchen 3-4mal tgl. Tagesdoses von 6 Filmtbl. bzw. 4 Zäpf. sollen nicht überschritten werden.
Dosage instruction: 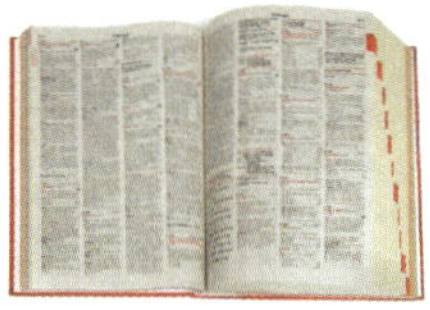	

DIALOG /ROLEPLAY

7 **Find two different medicines which your doctor often prescribes. Use the "Rote Liste" and write down dosage instructions for the patient in English. Write the brand names on a piece of paper and hand it to your teacher. The teacher will hand it out to one of your classmates who will ask you for dosage instructions.**

8 **Write a dialog with a partner. Complete the speech bubbles:**

Mr. Benton is leaving Dr. Millman's consulting room. His diagnosis is cystitis. Dr. Millman has prescribed an antibiotic called Cotrim forte® Hexal. Sarah (medical assistant) is leading Mr. Benton to the reception to print out the prescription.

MFA übergibt Patient das Antibiotikumrezept und teilt mit, dass man es unten in der Apotheke bekommt.

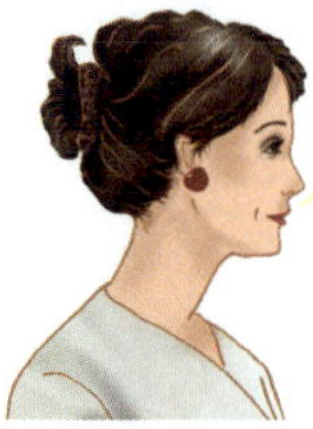

Patient äußert, dass er hofft, dass es schnell hilft, da er solche Schmerzen hat.

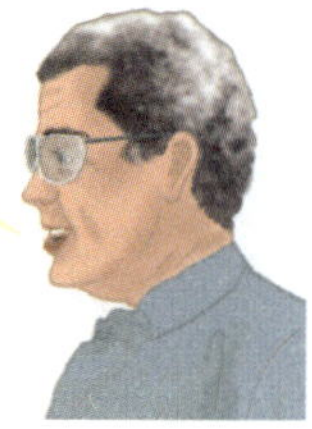

MFA macht ihm Mut, indem sie ihm mitteilt, dass das Antibiotikum meist schnell die Symptome lindert.

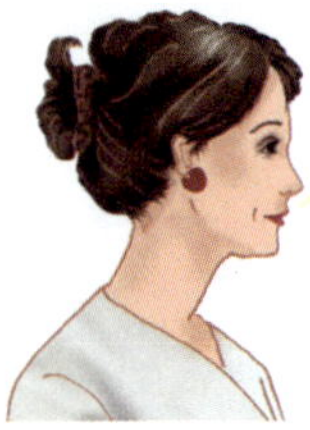

....

....

Patient ist froh das zu hören und fragt, ob er das Mittel absetzen kann, sobald er schmerzfrei ist.

....

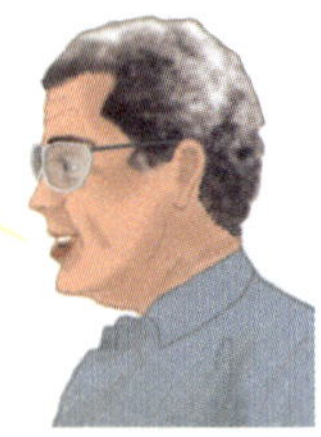

MFA betont, dass es wichtig ist, das Antibiotikum unbedingt nach Anweisung des Arztes einzunehmen. Um sicherzugehen, dass alle Keime in der Blase abgetötet werden, muss das Medikament solange eingenommen werden, wie der Arzt gesagt hat, nämlich vier Tage. Sonst besteht die Gefahr, dass die Blasenentzündung wiederkommt.

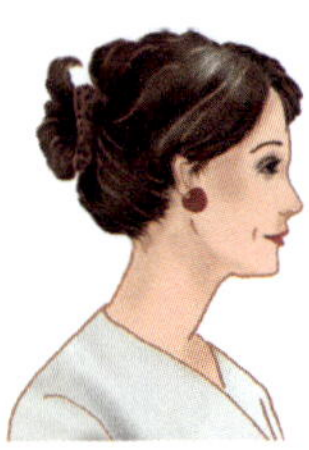

....

....

....

....

....

....

....

Patient fragt vorsichtshalber noch einmal nach, wie und wann er das Antibiotikum einnehmen soll.

....

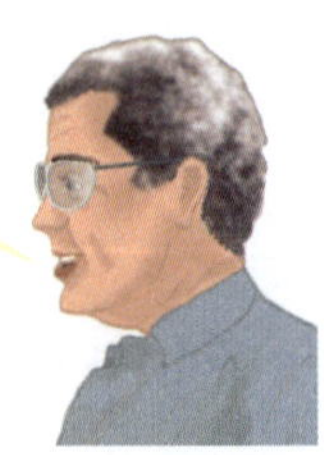

MFA schaut in der „Roten Liste“ nach und klärt denPatienten über die Dosierungsanleitung auf. Sie weist den Patienten darauf hin, dass er das Antibiotikum nicht mit Milch einnehmen darf, da es dann nicht richtig wirken kann. Er soll aber reichlich Wasser trinken, um die Bakterien aus der Blase zu spülen.

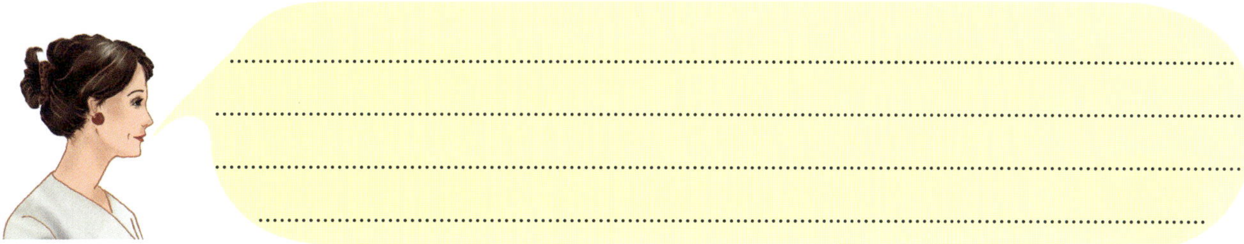

Patient fragt, ob er es auf nüchternen Magen nehmen muss.

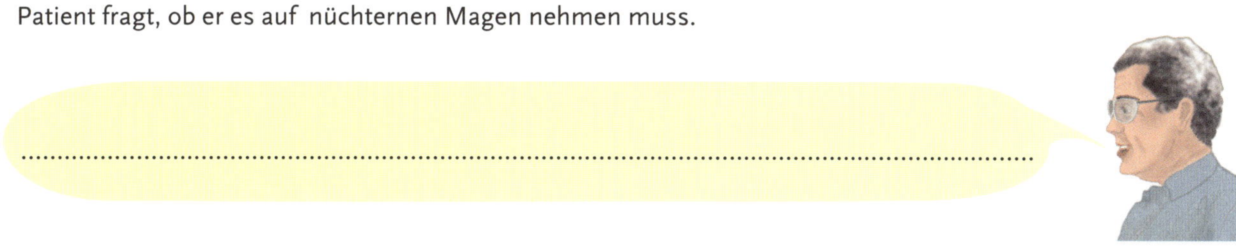

MFA schaut nochmals in der „Roten Liste“ nach und gibt Auskunft. Nach Beendigung der Einnahme soll sich der Patient zur Urinkontrolle wieder in der Praxis vorstellen.

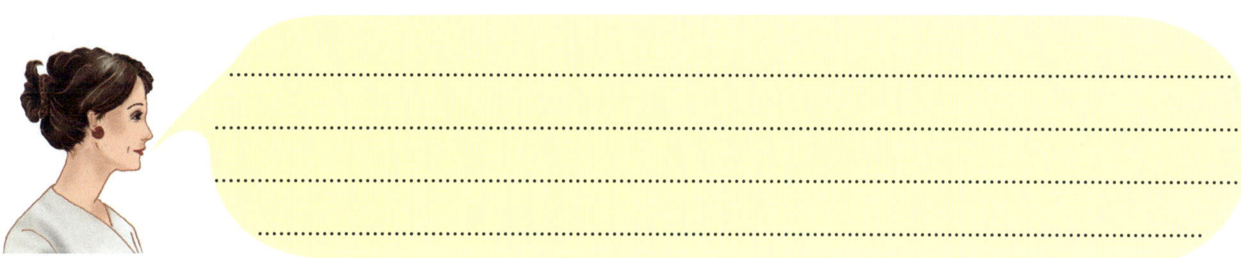

Patient bedankt sich bei der MFA und fragt nach einem Kontrolltermin.

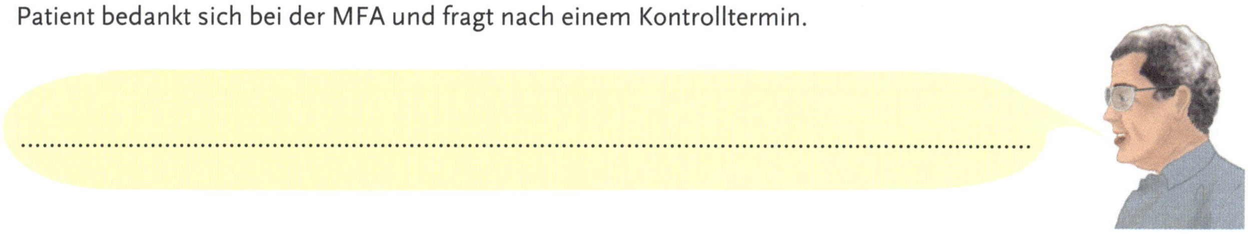

MFA schlägt Patient einen Termin am Donnerstagmorgen um 9:15 Uhr vor.

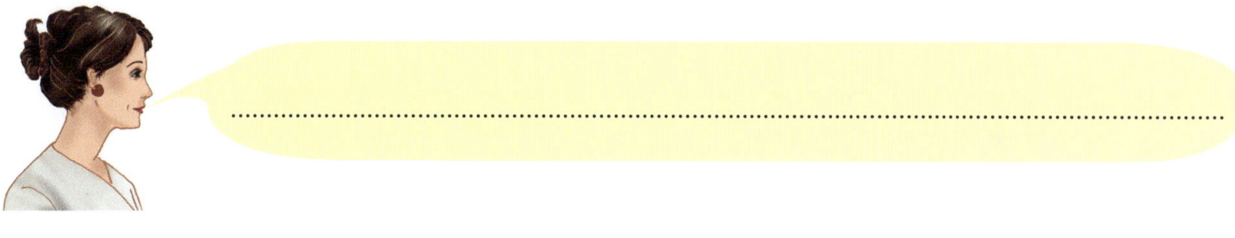

Dem Patient passt der Termin. Er wünscht der MFA einen schönen Tag.

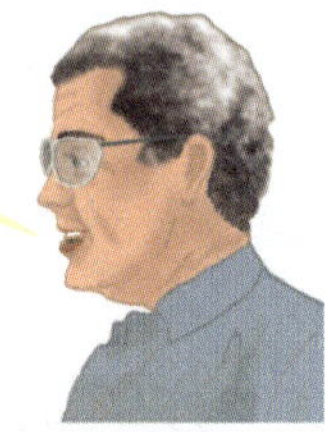

....

MFA wünscht gute Besserung und verabschiedet sich.

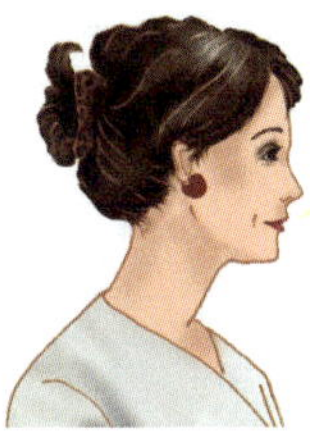

....

Antibiotics CRISS CROSS

9 **Fill in the crossword puzzle:**

Across

2. breathing organs
9. a medicine a woman uses to prevent pregnancy

Down

1. milk or food made from milk
3. a person who prepares and sells medicines
4. doctor
5. infection fighting drug
6. another word for medicine
7. cannot be harmed
8. you get ill or get a rash from a normally harmless substance
10. infection of the throat

13 24-Hour Urine Specimen

LISTENING Track 13

1 **Listen to the dialog and answer the following questions:**

- *What does the patient Mr. Scarano have to do?*
- *What is Perla's job?*
- *What questions does Mr. Scarano ask?*

READING

2 **Read the text. Check any new words in the vocabulary list or in a dictionary:**

For some examinations, like the creatinine clearance, the doctor needs a 24-hour urine specimen[1]. The patient has to collect the urine for a 24-hour period in special containers so that it can be analyzed in the laboratory later.

How to collect the urine:

You need to take your urine samples on the day before your doctor's appointment as follows:

- The first urine in the morning is not collected, it goes down the toilet.
- All further urine has to be collected in special containers. If you have to go to the toilet at night, this urine also has to be collected.
- The first urine from the next morning also goes into the container.
- Then you have to bring the containers filled with urine back to the doctor's practice.
- For some lab results, e.g. catecholamines (when pheochromocytoma[2] is suspected), the urine has to be mixed with hydrochloric acid[3]. This has to be added to the container after the first urine sample.

Example:

You have to go to the doctor's practice on Wednesday.
You get the urine containers on Monday BUT have to start collecting on Tuesday.

- On Monday evening you go to the toilet.
- On Tuesday morning you wake up and go to the toilet.
  -> Urine goes down the toilet.
- One hour later on Tuesday you have to go to the toilet again.
- At work you go to the toilet.
- On Wednesday morning you wake up and go to the toilet.
  -> This urine all goes into the container.

Important:

It is important that you collect the *whole* amount of urine. If you do not collect the whole amount, some lab results may be completely wrong.
You must only collect *urine* in these containers, nothing else!
If we take a blood sample today, you will have to bring the urine back within the next seven days, otherwise we have to take blood again. The urine has to be refrigerated[4] for this time.

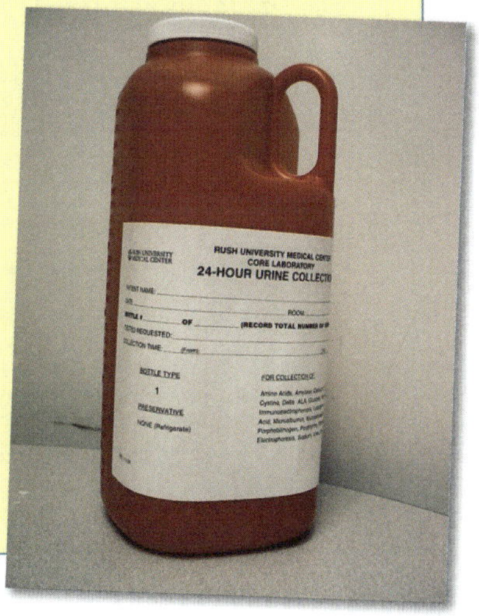

creatinine clearance, specimen, urine, laboratory, catecholamines, pheochromocytoma, hydrochloric acid

1 24-hour urine specimen – 24 h Sammelurin
2 pheochromocytoma – Phäochromozytom (Es handelt sich um einen Tumor, der Katecholamine produziert).
3 hydrochloric acid – Salzsäure
4 refrigerated – gekühlt

COMPREHENSION

3 Match the words with the correct explanation:

a) hydrochloric acid	[ ] normally found in the stomach as a digestive juice
b) 24-hour urine specimen	[ ] kind of kidney tumor that produces catecholamines
c) creatinine	[ ] patient has to collect his/her urine for a full day
d) pheochromocytoma	[ ] a test result which can be found in blood and urine

4 Fill in the gaps with the following words:

whole amount – blood creatinine level – 24-hour urine specimen – hydrochloric acid – 24 hours – in the morning – toilet – refrigerated – containers – urine

For the .... the patient has to collect his .... in special .... He/she has to collect for a period of .... He/she has to start .... , with the first urine going down the .... After collection, the urine has to be .... For some examinations the patient has to add .... to the containers. In order to ensure correct lab results, the .... of urine is needed. The .... must not be older than one week for the calculation of the creatinine clearance.

READING

5 Now read the dialog again and check any new vocabulary in the word list or in a dictionary:

Dr. Thaddäus wants a 24-hour urine specimen from the patient Marco Scarano. Mr. Scarano doesn't speak German, Dr. Thaddäus does not speak English, so Perla (medical assistant) has to talk to the patient and explain to him what the doctor wants.

Dr. T.: Perla, Herr Scarano bekommt noch einen Sammelurin mit Krea-Clearance, Elektrophorese und Gesamteiweiß. Sie können doch Englisch, machen Sie das mal.

Perla: Okay, ich werd´s ihm erklären.

Mr. Scarano: What did he say?!?

Perla: The doctor needs a 24-hour urine specimen to see how your kidneys work.

Mr. Scarano: What does he need? What is this specimen?

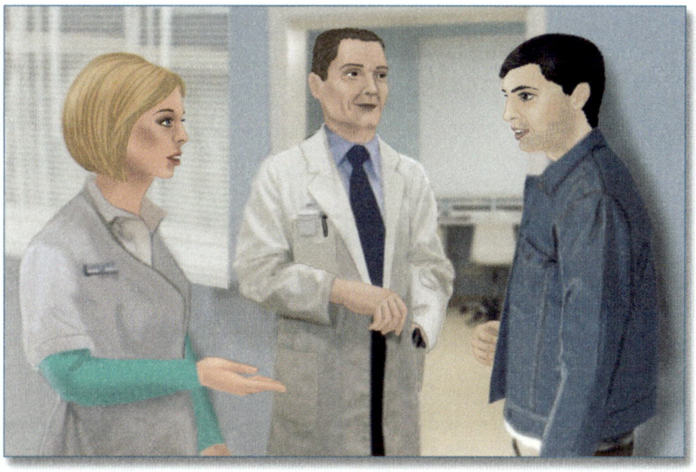

Perla: It means that you have to collect urine in special containers for 24 hours.

Mr. Scarano: Special containers? Where do I get them from? Why can't I collect it in a bottle?

Perla: You'll get these containers here in the practice, I'll give them to you later. You can't use any other bottles because they could lead to wrong lab results, e.g. if you use an empty coke bottle or a (nearly) empty glass of honey, you will have higher glucose results...

Mr. Scarano: Okay, I got it. And how do I have to collect my urine?

Perla gets the special containers.

Perla: These special containers will hold all of the urine you void in a 24-hour period and they must be refrigerated for this time. You must keep a record of the date and exact time when the collection begins, which should be at the second urination of the day. Then every time you pass water, day and night for the next 24-hours, you should urinate into a clean smaller container, which I'll give to you later, and add the urine to the larger container. The last sample included in the test period is the first urination of the next morning. When completed, you must bring the special containers into the practice and we will send it to our laboratory.

Mr. Scarano: So I have to start right after getting up in the morning?

Perla: No, the morning urine goes down the toilet. You start collecting from your second visit to the toilet.

Mr. Scarano: Do I have to take these containers with me to work?

Perla: Yes, I'm afraid you'll have to because we need the whole amount of urine. Or you can collect it over the weekend, e.g. from Sunday to Monday.

Mr. Scarano: Oh no, then I would prefer to take them to work... By the way, do I have to fill the containers completely? Then I would have to drink six liters!!

Perla: No, you should drink as usual. You don't have to fill up the containers completely. It is only important that you fill it with all the voided urine.

Mr. Scarano: What about my medicine? Can I take it as usual while collecting?

Perla: Yes, you can take your tablets as you usually do.

Mr. Scarano: OK, and when do I have to start collecting?

Perla: I will take a look in our appointment book.... Would next Wednesday, 9 o' clock, suit you? This means you would have to start collecting Tuesday. And you would have to come on an empty stomach because we will take a blood sample then, too.

Mr. Scarano: Yes, Wednesday would be fine. But why do you have to take a blood sample again? The last time was only about three weeks ago....

Perla: Because the blood creatinine result should not be older than one week for the calculation of the creatinine clearance. Therefore the laboratory needs both creatinine from blood and urine.

Mr. Scarano: Okay, then I'll get my containers and see you next Wednesday.

COMPREHENSION

5 **True or false? Correct false statements:**

	T/F
1. The doctor needs a 24-h-urine specimen to check the patient's liver function.	
2. Urine has to be collected for a full day.	
3. The urine has to be collected in special containers provided by the practice.	
4. The collected urine can be stored at room temperature.	
5. You should not pass the urine directly into the large container.	
6. You begin the collection with the first morning urine. The first morning urine of the following day goes down the toilet.	
7. Mr. Scarano does not have to collect urine at work.	
8. Perla also has to take a blood sample of Mr. Scarano to calculate the creatinine clearance.	
9. Mr. Scarano's appointment is on Thursday, so he has to start collecting on Monday.	

DIALOG / ROLEPLAY

6 **English role cards: Working with a partner, write a dialog using the following role cards:**

The doctor wants a 24–hour urine specimen from Naomi Miller. The medical assistant has to explain to Ms. Miller what she has to do and make an appointment with the patient.

Patient: Naomi Miller

Didn't understand what the doctor wants her to do.
Has no time on Tuesday.
Wants to know

- if she may take her tablets while collecting
- how much she has to drink
- why blood has to be taken again (last blood sample only two weeks ago)
- how she has to store the containers.

Medical assistant: Steffi Schmidt

The doctor wants her to explain to the patient how she has to collect the urine.
Next free appointment on Wednesday or Thursday.
MA has to explain / tell the patient

- why she has to use special containers
- when she has to start
- which urine goes down the toilet and which goes into the containers
- that she has to come on an empty stomach because a blood sample has to be taken again.

7 **German role cards – working with a partner, write a dialog using the following role cards: (for advanced students)**

Der Doktor braucht einen Sammelurin von Naomi Miller. Die MFA muss Frau Miller erklären, wie sie den 24h-Urin sammelt und mit ihr einen Termin vereinbaren.

Patient: Mrs. Naomi Miller

Hat nicht verstanden, was der Doktor von ihr wollte.
Sie hat keine Zeit am Dienstag. Sie ist Vollzeit berufstätig.
Möchte wissen:

- darf sie ihre Tabletten nehmen, während sie den 24h-Urin sammelt?
- wie viel sie trinken muss,
- warum noch mal Blut abgenommen werden muss (die letzte Blutentnahme war vor zwei Wochen),
- wie sie die Container verstauen soll,
- wie sie den Urin während ihrer Berufstätigkeit sammeln soll.

Medical assistant: Steffi Schmidt

Der Doktor möchte, dass die Arzthelferin der Patientin erklärt, wie sie den 24h-Urin sammeln muss.
Der nächste freie Termin wäre Mittwoch oder Donnerstag.
Sie muss der Patientin erklären/sagen,

- warum sie spezielle Container benutzen muss,
- wann sie beginnen muss,
- welcher Urin in die Toilette geht und welcher in die Container muss,
- dass sie nüchtern kommen muss, weil nochmal Blut abgenommen wird,
- wie sie die Uringewinnung mit ihrer Arbeit vereinbaren kann.

24-Hour Urine specimen WORD SEARCH

8 **Can you find 13 hidden words? Find the hidden message in the remaining letters.**

K	I	L	A	B	O	R	A	T	O	R	Y
D	N	E	Y	P	R	A	C	T	I	C	E
E	L	P	M	A	S	D	O	O	L	B	D
G	N	I	T	C	E	L	L	O	C	I	S
R	E	F	R	I	G	E	R	A	T	E	D
T	E	S	T	R	E	S	U	L	T	E	A
E	M	P	T	Y	S	T	O	M	A	C	H
C	O	N	T	A	I	N	E	R	U	S	S
N	E	M	I	C	E	P	S	E	R	T	L
K	L	R	A	M	O	U	N	T	I	O	E
P	E	R	S	L	N	H	E	N	N	R	H
E	T	A	L	U	C	L	A	C	E	E	K

....

....

....

....

....

....

....

Hidden message: ....

14 Prenatal Care

LISTENING Track 14

1 **Listen to the dialog and answer the following questions:**

- *What examination is being performed?*
- *Which does the medical assistant do?*

READING

2 **Read the text and check the vocabulary in bold print in the word list or in a dictionary:**

Prenatal care allows us to know how the baby is doing before birth, as well as how the mom is doing during ***pregnancy***. The aim is ***to detect*** problems early and ***to prevent*** them if possible.

Physical examinations consist of the mother's ***medical history, blood pressure, height*** and ***weight***, ***pelvic exam, ultrasound, cardiotocography, measuring the abdomen***, and blood and urine tests. The results are documented in a ***maternity record book***.

The blood can be tested for

- ***harmful*** infections like hepatitis B, syphilis and other ***sexually transmitted diseases***, HIV, toxoplasmosis, chlamydia
- antibodies against ***rubella (German measles)*** and ***chickenpox***. Both diseases can cause ***birth defects***.
- ***anemia*** (low red blood cell count), which leads to ***poor oxygen supply***. It could make you feel extremely tired and increases the risk of ***preterm labor***.
- your ***blood type*** and ***Rhesus factor***. Rh negative women need treatment to protect their babies from a dangerous blood problem.

The urine can be tested for

- urinary tract infections
- glucose, which could be a sign of diabetes and cause the baby ***to gain*** too much weight
- protein (which in combination with high blood pressure are symptoms of a pregnancy-related condition called ***preeclampsia***. This can lead to ***poor fetal growth***.)

Amniocentesis is a special prenatal test for women because they or their babies are at increased risk of certain problems.

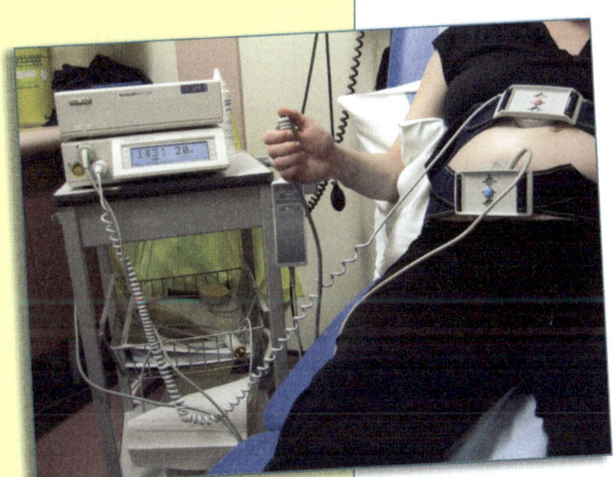

prenatal, pregnancy, cardiotocography, abdome, toxoplasmosis, chlamydia, anemia, oxygen, Rhesus factor, glucose, diabetes, protein, preeclampsia, amniocentesis

COMPREHENSION

3 **Answer the following questions and write the answers down:**

1. What is prenatal care?

....

....

....

2. What examinations/tests are done?

....

....

....

3. Name potentially harmful infections during pregnancy.

....

....

....

4. Why should anemia be treated?

....

....

5. Why is it important to find out the mother's blood type?

....

....

6. Why could glucose/protein positive urine be a problem?

....

....

....

4 **Fill in the gaps with the words below. Which word does not fit?** ....

abdomen – anemic – blood pressure – blood type – cardiotocography – diabetes – glucose – height – infections – overweight – prenatal care – Rhesus negative – takes blood – tiredness – ultrasound – urine sample – weight

.... is done to find out if the pregnant woman and her unborn baby are healthy. The medical assistant measures the ...., ... and .... of the pregnant patient. She also needs a .... from the patient to analyze if there is protein or .... in the urine. If it tests positive for sugar, this may be a sign of .... Then there is the risk that the unborn becomes .... The medical assistant also .... to find out if the patient is .... This can cause extreme .... in the mother and preterm labor. The blood is also tested for dangerous .... and .... If the pregnant woman is .... it may lead to serious blood problems in the baby. Later in the pregnancy, the .... is measured regularly. Pelvic exam and .... are both performed by the doctor.

Fetal Monitoring / Cardiotocography (CTG)

READING

5 **Read the text and check any vocabulary in a dictionary:**

In medicine (obstetrics[1]), cardiotocography is a technical recording[2] (-graphy) of the fetal ***heart rate*** (cardio-) and the ***uterine contractions*** (-toco-). This test is typically done in the third trimester of the pregnancy to identify fetal distress[3]. It is also done during childbirth when the woman has labor pains[4]. The recordings are done by two separate sensors (transducers), one working with ultrasound for the ***measurement*** of the fetal heartbeat and the other one for the uterine contractions. They are ***taped*** to the ***abdominal wall*** of the pregnant woman. The CTG reading is ***printed*** on paper and/or ***stored*** on a computer. The upper line indicates[5] the fetal heart rate and the lower line the uterine contractions.

1 obstetrics – Geburtshilfe
2 recording – Aufzeichnung
3 distress – Leid, Schmerz
4 labor pains – Wehen
5 to indicate – anzeigen

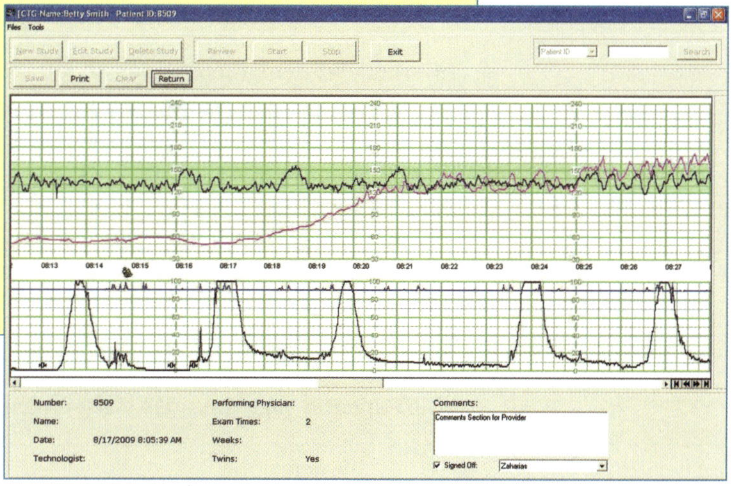

CTG CRISS CROSS

6 **Fill in the puzzle:**

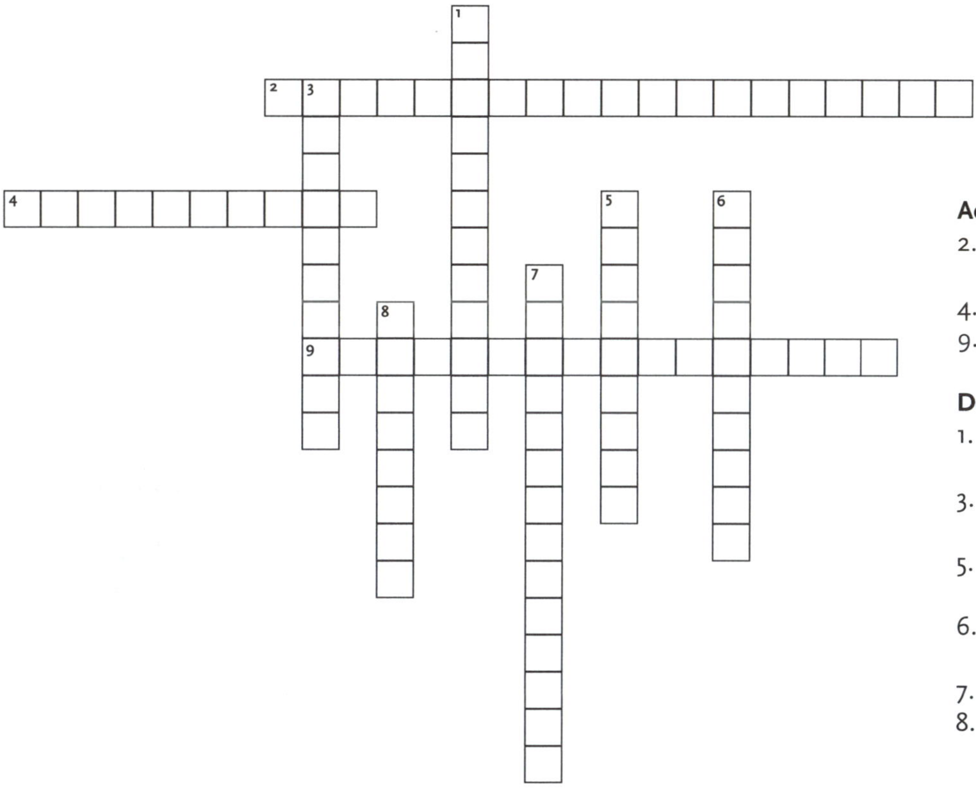

Across

2. What are the cramps in the lower abdomen called?
4. A CTG works with...
9. What does "CTG" stand for?

Down

1. What do you call a doctor who specializes in prenatal care?
3. What has to be attached to the stomach?
5. The lower line ... the uterine contractions.
6. While giving birth the woman has...
7. What does the CTG record?
8. The woman is ... when she comes for the CTG.

DIALOG / ROLEPLAY

7 **Write a dialog with a partner. Complete the speech bubbles.**
If you finish early, also write a dialog for what has been done before the CTG (taking blood, blood pressure, urine check).

Shari Amoah, a 30 week pregnant woman, comes for a check-up into your practice. First you (medical assistant) ask for her maternity record book to document the results. After taking her blood pressure, taking a blood sample and asking her for a urine sample, you now have to record a CTG. It's the first CTG the pregnant woman has had.

MFA erklärt der Patientin, dass heute zusätzlich ein CTG bei ihr aufgezeichnet wird. Sie begleiten die Patientin ins Untersuchungszimmer.

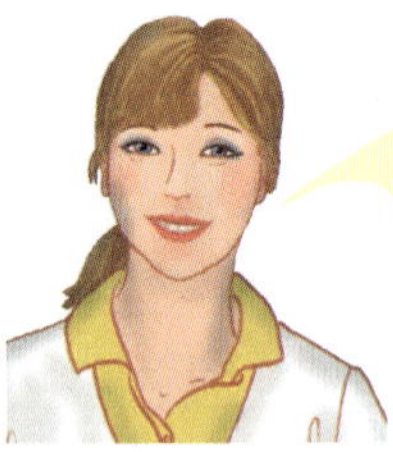

Die Patientin sagt, dass das bisher nicht gemacht wurde und sie das nicht kennt.

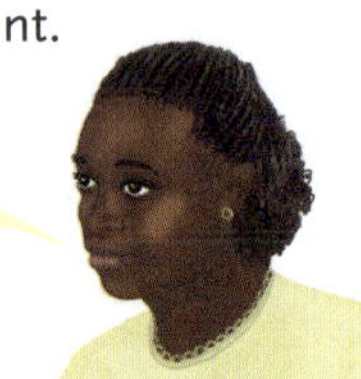

MFA erklärt, dass das CTG mit Ultraschall die Herztöne des Fötus und die Wehentätigkeit aufzeichnet.

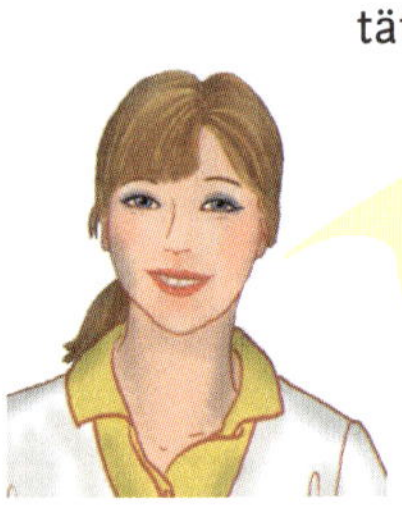

Die Patientin fragt, wofür diese Untersuchung gemacht wird.

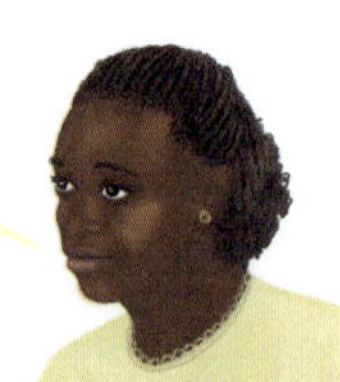

MFA erläutert, dass diese Untersuchung kontrolliert, ob das Herz des Babys richtig schlägt und wie es bei Kontraktionen, z.B. Wehen oder Husten, schlägt.

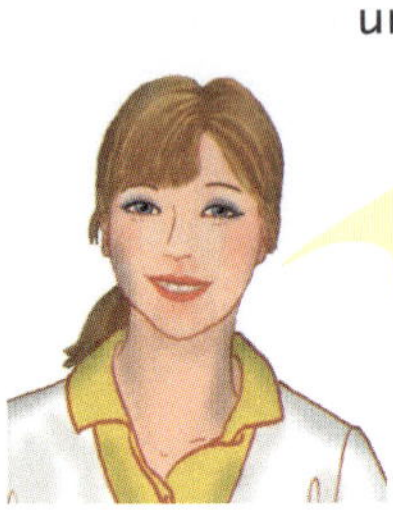

Die Patientin äußert, dass sie nicht weiß, was sie tun muss.

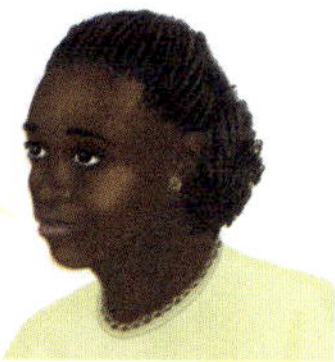

MFA weist sie an, sich auf die Liege zu legen und den Bauch frei zu machen.

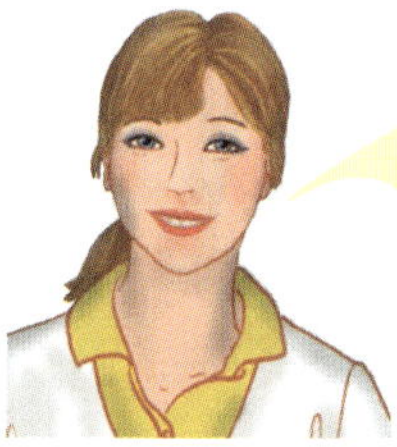

MFA klärt über ihre nächsten Schritte auf. Sie befestigt den Wehenschreiber und den Schallkopf für die Herztätigkeit am Bauch der Patientin und fordert die Patientin auf, sich zu entspannen.

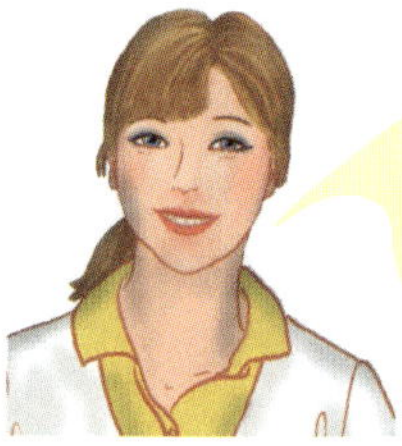

Die Patientin fragt, wie lange es dauern wird.

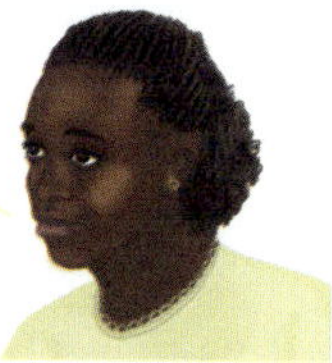

MFA informiert, dass es ca. 20 Minuten dauern wird, wenn das Gerät gut aufzeichnet.

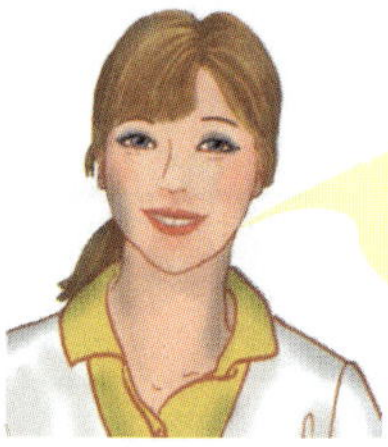

Die Patientin möchte wissen, was die Linien bedeuten.

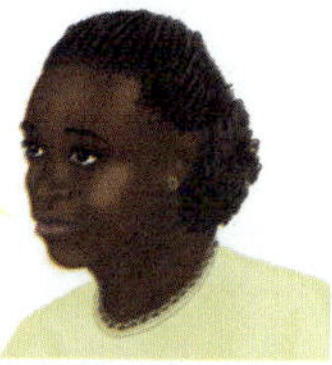

MFA erklärt, dass die obere Linie die Herztöne und die untere Linie die Wehentätigkeit anzeigt.

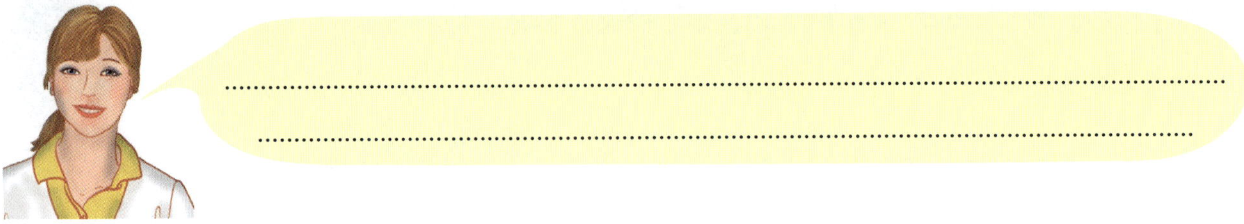

Nach 20 Minuten entfernt die MFA die Schallköpfe und sagt, dass sie das Ergebnis noch dem Doktor vorlegt und der Patientin dann Bescheid gibt, ob sie gehen kann. In der Zwischenzeit kann die Patientin im Wartezimmer Platz nehmen.

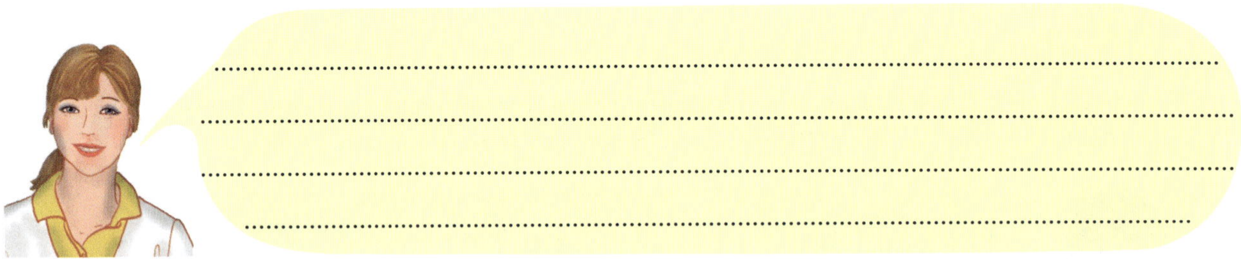

CTG-CRYPTOGRAM

8 **Which numbers represent which letters?**

A	B	C	D	E	F	G	H	I	J	K	L	M	N	O	P	Q	R	S	T	U	V	W	X	Y	Z
			7				15	13									11	2			16				

_H_ (19 15 21)   _____ (18 21 19 6 26)   H__RT (15 21 6 11 19)   R___ (11 6 19 21)   __D (6 14 7)   _H_ (19 15 21)   ___RI__ (10 19 21 11 13 14 21)

____R___I__S (24 8 14 19 11 6 24 19 13 8 14 2)   _R_ (6 11 21)   R___RD_D (11 21 24 8 11 7 21 7)   _I_H (12 13 19 15)   ___R_S___D (10 26 19 11 6 2 8 10 14 7)

VI_ (16 13 6)   _R__SD___R (19 11 6 14 2 7 10 24 21 11)   __ (8 14)   _H_ (19 15 21)   S______ (2 19 8 3 6 24 15)

15 Fecal Occult Blood Test (FOBT)

LISTENING Track 15

1 **Listen to the dialog and answer the following questions:**

- *What kind of test does the patient have to do?*
- *What is the test for?*
- *How does the patient have to prepare?*
- *How do you do the test?*

READING

2 **Read the dialog and check the words in bold print in the vocabulary list or in a dictionary:**

Mrs. Simpson is 51 years old and consults an internist for a check-up. The medical assistant measures her blood pressure, takes blood and hands her a FOB test. Now she has to explain the test to Mrs. Simpson.

(MA = Medical Assistant   Pat. = Patient)

MA: Mrs. Simpson, this is a test to find out whether you have ***hidden*** blood in your ***stool***. You have reached an age where this test is ***recommended*** as a ***preventive medical check-up***. Positive results can be a sign of ***polyps***, ***ulcers*** and even ***colon cancer***. Early detection[1] means a better chance of a ***cure*** because of possible early treatment.

Pat.: Oh, that's a sensible[2] test. Do I have to consider[3] anything in particular?

MA: Very good question. Yes, you have to prepare for the test. Three days before the test and while collecting ***stool samples*** you mustn't eat ***raw meat*** or too much vitamin C. Stop taking aspirin if you take any.

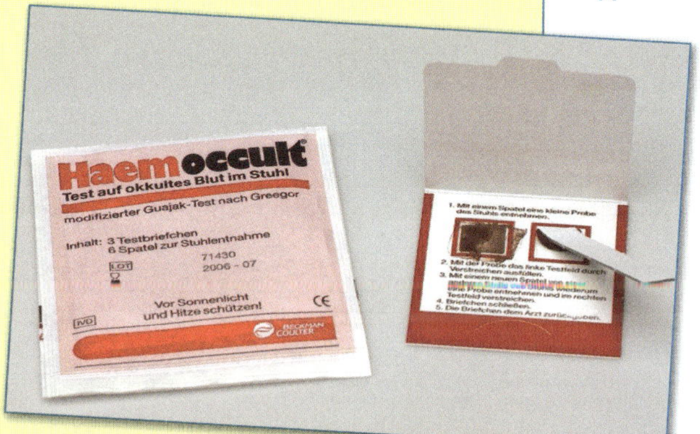

Pat.: And how do I have to do this test?

MA: You have to collect three test samples of your stool from three following ***bowel movements***. First open the side which states "für den Patienten", that means "for the patient". Don't open the other side, because it's only for the doctor. Take a piece of newspaper and place it under the toilet seat because the stool mustn't fall into the water. After that you take one of the applicator sticks[4] and take a (***pea size***) bit of your stool and ***smear*** it on one of the test fields. Then take a second sample with a new applicator stick from a different ***site*** of the stool. Now close the ***cover***. Write down your name and the date of the sample. Collect all three samples and take them back to us.

Pat.: Okay, thank you.

MA: No problem, if you have any questions, please give us a call.

Pat.: Thank you again. I will bring it back in three days.

Fecal Occult Blood Test ,
polyp,
ulcer,
bowel movement,
applicator sticks

1 detection – Feststellen, Entdecken
2 sensible – sinnvoll
3 to consider – beachten
4 applicator stick – Spatel

COMPREHENSION

3 **True or false? Correct false statements.**

	T/F
1. This test is done to find out if you have urine in your stool.	
2. The preventive medical check-up is for men over 45 years.	
3. Early detection means a better chance of getting sick again.	
4. You have to prepare for the test seven days beforehand.	
5. You must not eat turnip, raw meat or pasta.	
6. You have to take three subsequent test samples.	
7. Open the cover on the side "für den Patienten", which means " for the patient".	
8. Take a piece of newspaper and place it over the toilet seat because the stool should fall into the water.	
9. Take one of the applicator sticks and take your whole stool and smear it on one of the test fields.	
10. Collect all three samples and take them back to the practice as soon as possible.	
11. A medical cause for a positive test result could be influenza.	
12. Diet has an influence on the test.	

4 **Fill in the gaps with the words below:**

cover – raw – test fields – prepare – name – collect – für den Patienten – applicator sticks – occult blood – smear – vitamin C – test samples – only for the patient – date

1. This test is to find out if you have .... in your stool.
2. You have to .... for the test three days beforehand.
3. You must not eat .... meat or too much ....

4. You have to take three subsequent .... of your stool.
5. Open the .... on the side which states " .... ", that means " .... ".
6. Take one of the .... and take a bit of your stool (pea size) and .... it on one of the ....
7. Write down your .... and the .... of the sample.
8. .... all three samples and take them back to the practice as soon as possible.

5 **Now translate the above sentences into German:**

1. Dieser Test ....
2. Sie müssen ....
3. Sie dürfen ....
4. Sie müssen ....
5. Öffnen Sie ....
6. Sie nehmen ....
7. Notieren Sie ....
8. Sammeln Sie ....

ROLEPLAY / DIALOG

6 **Write a dialog with a partner. Complete the speech bubbles.**
Rehearse and be prepared to act it out in class.

Mr. Wellings from New Zealand, aged 47, has come to see Dr. Gastric today because of irregular bowel movements sometimes combined with abdominal pain. Dr. Gastric has just taken his medical history and examined him. The doctor is asking you to take blood and give the patient a fecal occult blood test to do at home. Now it is your job to give him instructions how to do the test. You inform him that all instructions are written down on the test.

Der Patient äußert, dass er die Anleitung auf den Testbriefen leider nicht versteht, weil sein Deutsch noch schlecht ist und bittet die MFA um Hilfe.

....
....
....
....

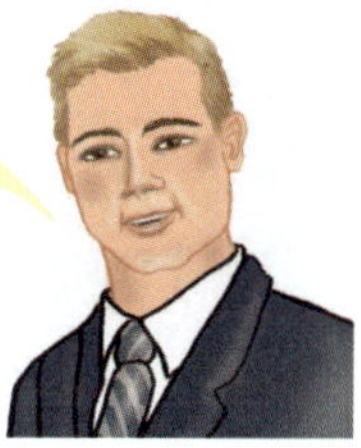

MFA bejaht seine Bitte und entschuldigt sich dafür, dass sie vergessen hat, dass der Patient englischsprachig ist.

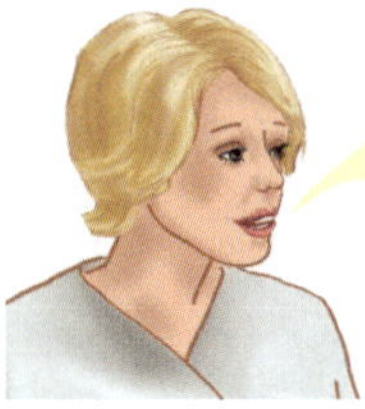

MFA erklärt und demonstriert mithilfe des Testbriefes, wie er die Testproben gewinnt, die Toilette präpariert, wo er seine Proben platzieren soll, auch wie er mit dem Spatel umzugehen hat, und dass er Namen und Datum auf dem Briefchen notieren soll.

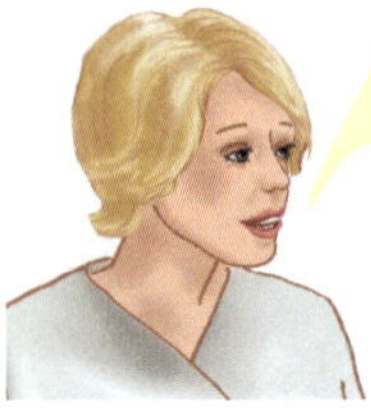

Der Patient fragt, ob er noch etwas zu beachten hat.

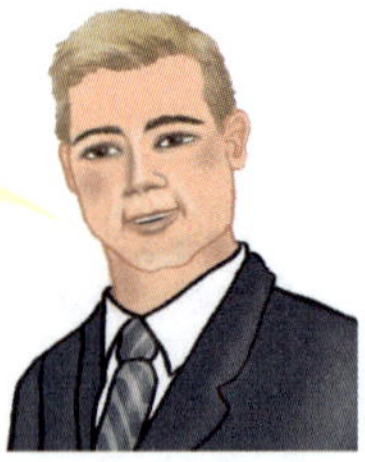

MFA erklärt, dass er drei Tage vor dem Test keine Radieschen, keinen Meerrettich, keine Rüben, nicht soviel Vitamin C und kein blutiges oder rotes Fleisch essen darf, weil dadurch das Testergebnis verfälscht werden könnte.

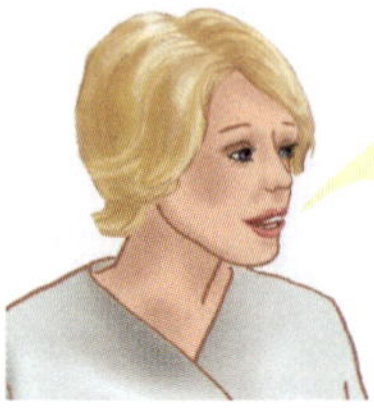

Der Patient bedankt sich.

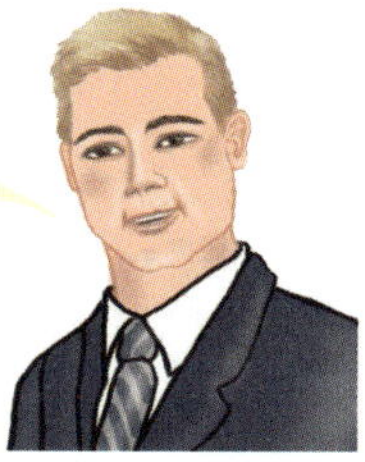

MFA bietet an, dass der Patient, wenn er Probleme oder Fragen hat, gerne anrufen darf.

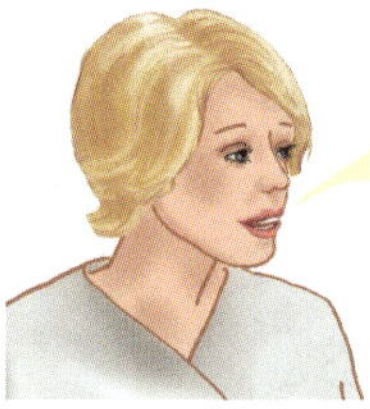

Der Patient hat noch eine Frage, er wüsste gerne, wofür dieser Test gemacht wird.

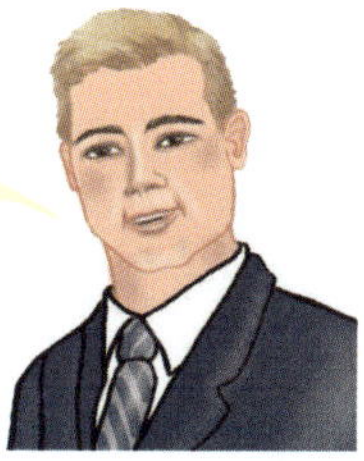

MFA erklärt, dass der Test den Stuhl auf verstecktes Blut untersucht und damit ein eventueller Darmkrebs, Geschwüre oder Polypen erkannt werden können. Dies erhöht seine Heilungschancen. Dieser Test wird auch innerhalb der Krebsvorsorge bei Männern über 45 Jahren gemacht.

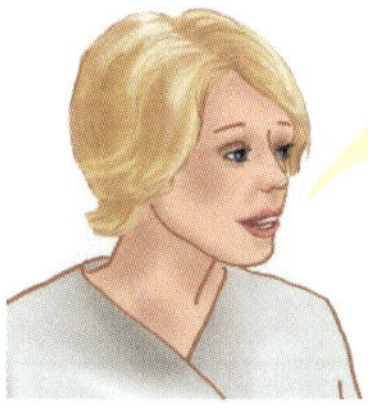

Patient findet es toll, dass es so einen Test gibt, bedankt sich noch einmal und sagt, dass er die Proben in drei Tagen wieder bringt.

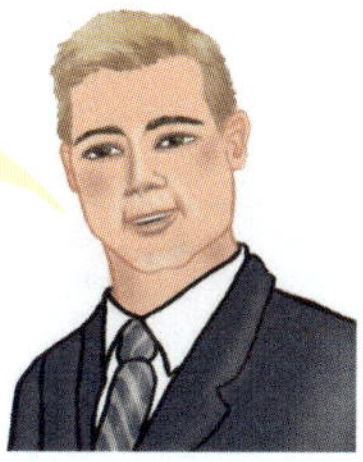

ROLECARDS (for advanced students)

7 **Prepare a role play from the directions printed below. Rehearse and be prepared to act it out in class.**

Medical assistant Jenny

Mrs. Shell kommt aus dem Sprechzimmer von Dr. Colon. Im Rahmen der Krebsvorsorge soll Mrs. Shell einen Test auf okkultes Blut im Stuhl durchführen. Sie haben die Aufgabe, ihr die Vorbereitung und Durchführung des Stuhltests zu erklären.
Erklären Sie ihr die diätetischen Maßnahmen, die Mrs. Shell einhalten muss.
Erklären Sie Mrs. Shell die Testdurchführung.
Mrs. Shell zeigt sich nicht immer einsichtig. Ihre Gewohnheiten sind nicht mit der Testvorbereitung vereinbar. Versuchen Sie Ihr Bestes, um Mrs. Shell dazu zu bringen, den Test korrekt durchzuführen.

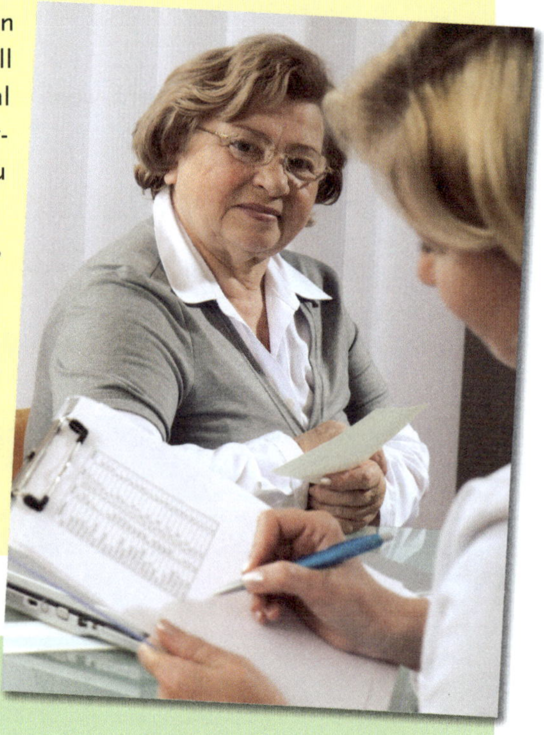

Patient Mrs. Shell, 70 years old

Ihnen ging im Gespräch mit dem Arzt alles zu schnell. Deshalb fragen Sie jetzt noch einmal bei der MFA zu folgenden Punkten nach:

- warum der Test durchgeführt wird
- was genau damit untersucht werden soll

Die vorbereitenden Maßnahmen sind gegen ihre Gewohnheiten. Sie essen gerne Fleisch und Weißbrot, Gemüse, Obst und Vollkornprodukte hingegen ungern. Stuhlgang haben Sie deshalb auch nur ca. alle drei Tage.
Mit Kopfschmerzen haben Sie regelmäßig zu tun und behandeln diese in der Regel immer mit einigen Aspirintabletten.
Bei der Probengewinnung zeigen Sie sich nicht immer einsichtig.

Word Search FOB-Test

8 **Can you find 17 hidden words?**
Find the hidden message in the remaining letters:

T	E	P	R	E	V	E	N	T	I	O	N	U	G	C
E	O	A	T	O	P	R	E	V	E	N	T	L	I	A
S	V	E	R	C	H	E	C	K	U	P	S	C	Q	N
T	X	E	E	L	H	E	A	L	T	H	Y	E	A	C
F	O	G	C	V	Y	H	Q	U	O	M	D	R	E	E
I	U	S	N	D	E	D	N	E	M	M	O	C	E	R
E	W	B	A	I	T	C	E	L	L	O	C	Y	Z	C
L	P	A	C	V	P	M	E	T	N	E	D	D	I	H
D	T	V	N	Z	S	Y	H	Z	E	V	F	E	L	E
Y	I	R	O	R	K	W	L	P	I	C	P	V	I	C
A	P	P	L	I	C	A	T	O	R	S	T	I	C	K
M	J	I	O	O	Y	D	C	I	P	O	A	I	T	U
B	O	C	C	U	L	T	B	L	O	O	D	E	O	P
B	O	W	E	L	M	O	V	E	M	E	N	T	P	N
E	L	P	M	A	S	L	O	O	T	S	I	T	E	I

Hidden Message:

16 Colonoscopy

LISTENING Track 16

1 **Listen to the dialog and answer the following questions:**

- *What is Ms. Simpson tested for?*
- *What does the medical assistant have to do?*

READING

2 **Read the following text and check words in bold print in the vocabulary list or in a dictionary:**

colonoscopy, large intestine, colonoscope, caecum, biopsy, diarrhea, ulcerative colitis, polyps, coagulation, laxatives, sedative

1 to insert – einführen
2 advisable – ratsam
3 persistant – andauernd
4 to confirm – bestätigen
5 coagulation – Gerinnung
6 lining – Schleimhaut
7 to remove – entfernen
8 to accompany – begleiten

A ***colonoscopy*** is a test where the doctor looks into the ***colon***, also called ***large intestine***. A ***colonoscope*** is a thin, flexible telescope that is inserted[1] into the ***anus*** and then pushed all the way round the colon as far as the ***caecum***. It has a light and a side channel so that a sample (***biopsy***) can be taken.

A colonoscopy is advisable[2] if you have the following symptoms:

- bleeding from the anus
- ***lower abdominal pain***
- persistent[3] ***diarrhea***

Conditions which can be confirmed[4] are for example:

- ulcerative colitis
- Crohn's disease
- colon ***polyps***
- colon cancer

In Germany a colonoscopy is advised as a preventive medical check-up for adults aged over 50.

Procedure:

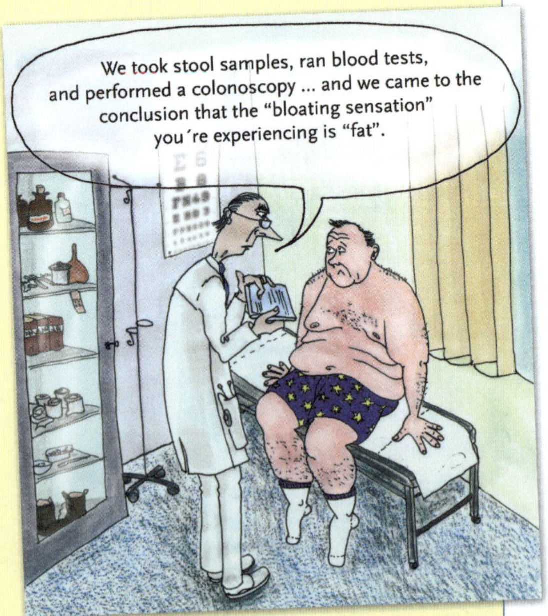

Before the test is done the patient has to fill in and sign a medical history form. Also, a blood sample is taken to check the patient's coagulation[5].

The colon has to be empty so that the doctor can get a clear view. Therefore the patient has to take ***laxatives*** and will be given instructions on his/her diet a few days before the test such as not to eat cereals, pulses or certain vegetables. On the day of the test the patient will usually be given a ***sedative*** to help him/her to relax. He/she lies on his side on a couch. The colonoscope is then gently pushed into the anus. The doctor can see the pictures on a monitor and inspect the lining[6] of the colon. For a better view, air is blown into the colon which may make the patient feel ***bloated*** and ***pass wind***. Taking biopsies is painless for the patient. They are sent to the lab for testing. If polyps are found they are directly removed[7].

A colonoscopy normally takes 20 – 50 minutes. After the test the patient needs some time to rest ***to recover*** from the sedative. The patient also needs somebody to accompany[8] him/her as the patient will feel ***drowsy*** and sleepy and is, of course, not allowed to drive.

COMPREHENSION

3 **Match the words with their definition:**

1. colonoscopy	a. liquid feces
2. anus	b. medicine that calms you or makes you sleep
3. biopsy	c. a small unhealthy growth of tissue inside the colon
4. diarrhea	d. intestines/colon full of air/gas
5. polyp	e. to force air out of the anus
6. laxative	f. a test where you look into a patient's large intestine
7. sedative	g. sleepy and not able to think clearly
8. bloated	h. the body part where feces leave the body
9. to pass wind	j. tissue sample
10. to recover	k. medicine to cure you from constipation
11. to feel drowsy	l. to become well again

4 **Answer the following questions:**

1. Describe the route the colonoscope takes through the body.

   ....

   ....

2. What are the indications for a colonoscopy? List the symptoms:

   ....

   ....

   ....

3. How does the patient have to prepare for the test?

   ....

   ....

   ....

   ....

4. What can happen to the patient when air is blown into his colon?

   ....

   ....

5. What happens to the samples of the biopsy?

   ....

   ....

6. What happens if the doctor detects a polyp?

   ....

   ....

7. Why does the patient need to bring another person to accompany him/her?

   ....

5 **Please complete the conversation below with the following words:**

appointment – allowed – breakfast – colonoscopy – drinking – drowsy – examination – sedative – laxative – muesli – prescription – pulses – vegetables – waiting-room

6 **Put the conversation into the correct order and then listen to the CD to check your answers:**

a. Ms. S: The doctor told me I should make an appointment for a ....

b. MA: No, you mustn't. For about 24 hours you are not .... to drive, work or make any important decisions because you'll feel .... from the sedative. We will call you a taxi or somebody should pick you up.

c. Ms. S: Okay, now I think I know everything. Thank you for your help.
MA: Then here is your .... and your .... slip.

d. MA: Good morning. How can I help you?

e. MA: On the morning before the test you may have .... as normal. You then need to stop eating. At 2 p.m. you should start .... "Endofalk"® and should have drunk it all by 8 p.m. to empty your intestines.

f. MA: Did the doctor tell you how to take your .... "Endofalk"®?
Ms. S: Yes he did, but I'm not sure if I understood everything.

g. Ms. S: My name is Simpson. I have an appointment with the doctor.

h. MA: Would 20th of June at 9 a.m. suit you?
Ms. S: Yes, that would be fine.

i. MA: No, you may not. Seven days before the .... you have to stop eating cereals. And 14 days beforehand you should stop eating .... like peas, beans and .... like tomatoes or peppers.

j. Ms. S: Does the examination hurt?

k. Ms. S: Can I drive home by car after that?

l. MA: What do you think you didn't understand?
Ms. S: When do I have to start taking "Endofalk"®?

m. Ms. S: May I eat .... ?

n. MA: It could hurt a little, but you can get a ....

o. MA: Oh yes, Ms. Simpson. Please take a seat in the ...., the doctor will call you.

DIALOG / ROLEPLAY

7 **Write a dialog with a partner. Complete the speech bubbles without looking at the text above:**

Ms. Simpson would like to see Dr. Steiner (gastroenterologist) because she detected blood in her stool. After taking her medical history and some examinations, Dr. Steiner decides to do a colonoscopy. Your job is to give her instructions on how to prepare for this examination.

MFA begrüßt Ms. Simpson und fragt, ob sie ihr helfen kann.

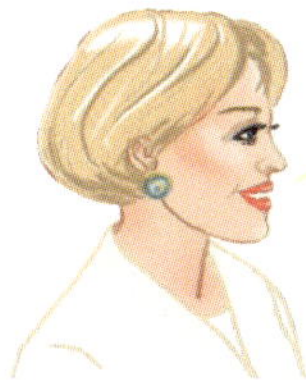

....

Ms. Simpson sagt, dass sie einen Termin hat.

....

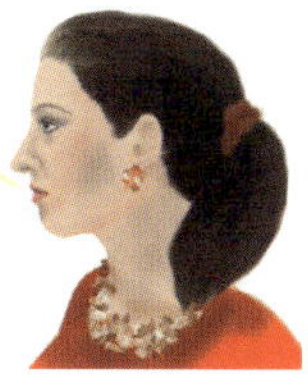

MFA bittet Ms. Simpson im Wartezimmer Platz zu nehmen, bis der Doktor sie ruft.

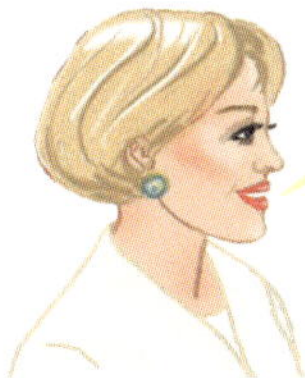

....

....

After the consultation

Ms. Simpson sagt, dass sie einen Termin für eine Koloskopie machen soll.

....

....

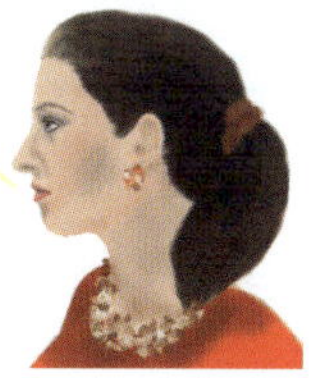

MFA fragt, ob der 20. Juni um 9:00 Uhr recht ist.

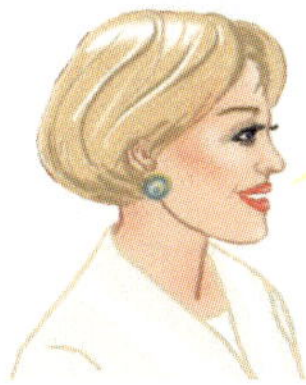

....

Ms. Simpson sagt, dass sie mit dem Termin einverstanden ist.

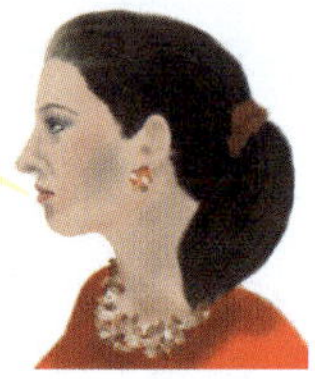

MFA fragt, ob der Doktor ihr erklärt hat, wie sie ihr Abführmittel Endofalk® nehmen soll.

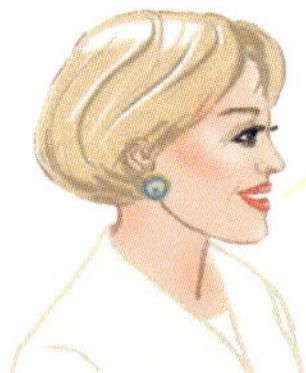

Ms. Simpson sagt, dass der Doktor es ihr erklärt hat, sie ist aber nicht sicher, ob sie alles verstanden hat.

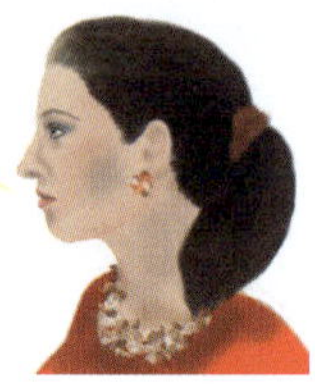

MFA fragt, was sie glaubt, nicht verstanden zu haben.

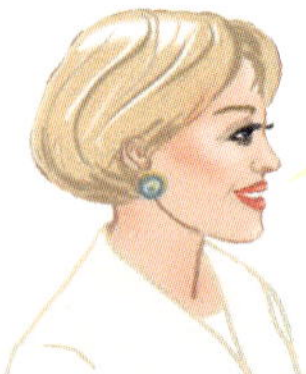

Ms. Simpson fragt, wann sie mit der Einnahme beginnen soll.

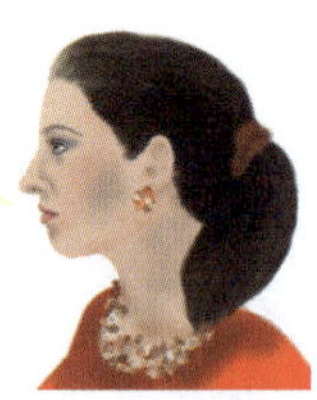

MFA erklärt, dass sie am Vortag normal frühstücken, dann aber nichts mehr essen darf. Gegen 14:00 soll sie mit der Einnahme des Abführmittels beginnen und bis 20:00 alles getrunken haben.

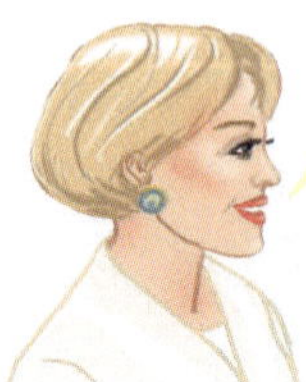

Ms. Simpson fragt, ob sie Müsli essen darf.

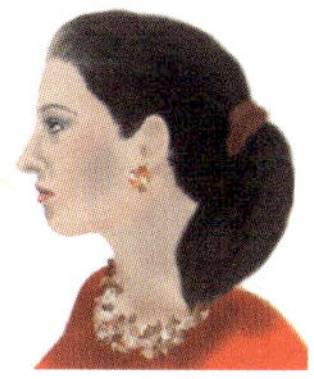

MFA sagt, dass sie kein Müsli essen darf. Sieben Tage vor der Untersuchung darf sie keine Körner mehr zu sich nehmen und 14 Tage vorher keine Hülsenfrüchte wie z.B. Erbsen, Bohnen und Gemüse wie Paprika oder Tomaten essen.

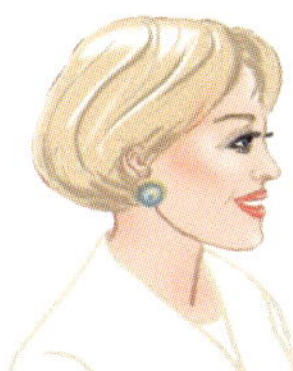

Ms. Simpson fragt, ob ihr die Untersuchung Schmerzen bereiten wird.

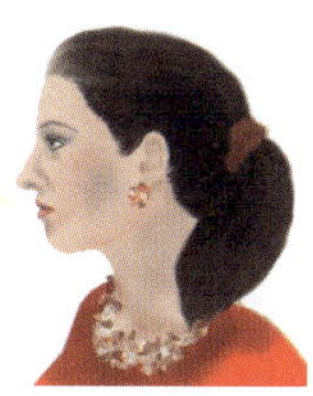

MFA sagt, dass es ein wenig schmerzen könnte, aber dass die Möglichkeit besteht, ein Beruhigungsmittel zu bekommen.

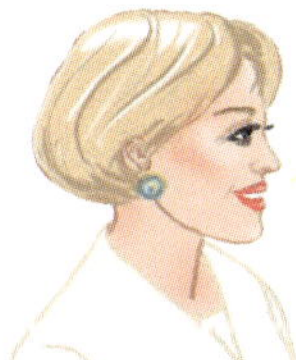

Ms. Simpson fragt, ob sie danach mit dem Auto fahren darf.

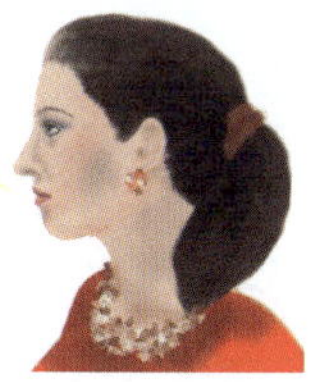

MFA verneint. Sie erklärt, dass sie 24 Stunden lang nicht alleine Auto fahren oder arbeiten darf. Sie sollte auch keine wichtigen Entscheidungen treffen, da sie vom Beruhigungsmittel benommen ist. MFA sagt, dass ein Taxi gerufen würde oder jemand Ms. Simpson abholen müsste.

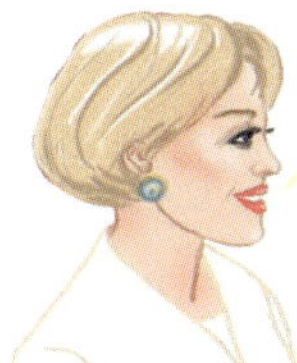

Ms. Simpson bedankt sich für die Informationen und verabschiedet sich.

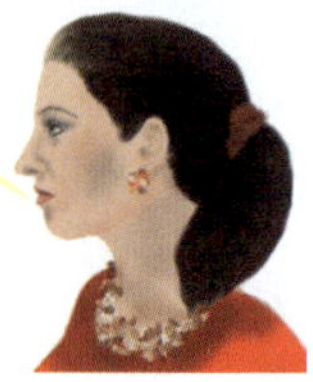

MFA antwortet und verabschiedet sich ebenfalls.

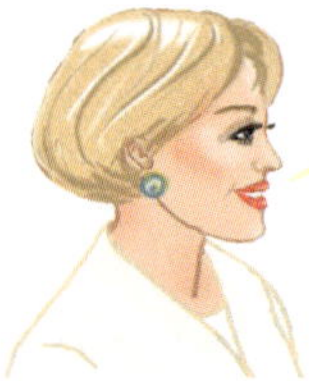

Colonoscopy WORD SEARCH

8 **Can you find the 23 hidden words?**

Y	Y	B	U	B	D	A	L	T	R	M	Y	N	D	S
W	R	W	R	R	I	A	N	E	H	P	W	O	E	E
S	C	O	O	E	X	O	V	U	O	F	D	I	T	C
E	E	W	T	A	A	O	P	C	S	O	I	T	A	E
C	S	S	T	S	C	K	S	S	D	Y	A	A	O	F
Y	D	I	L	E	I	O	F	Z	Y	V	R	P	L	C
D	V	A	R	U	N	H	B	A	U	B	R	I	B	K
E	R	U	T	O	P	D	L	J	S	Q	H	T	T	N
B	J	F	L	L	N	A	N	A	N	T	E	S	I	L
V	M	O	O	U	B	N	M	I	C	S	A	N	S	E
B	C	E	R	E	A	L	S	U	W	I	Z	O	S	D
I	N	T	E	S	T	I	N	E	S	S	D	C	U	D
I	L	S	E	U	M	P	O	L	Y	P	S	E	E	I
H	F	R	G	R	G	F	W	K	J	B	C	A	M	E
O	E	V	I	T	A	D	E	S	N	B	Z	J	P	T

17 Oral Glucose Tolerance Test (OGTT)

LISTENING Track 17

1 **Listen to the dialog and answer the following questions:**

- *What test should be performed and why?*
- *What instructions does the medical assistant give?*

READING

2 **Read the text and check the words in bold print in the vocabulary list or in a dictionary:**

The OGTT is ***usually*** used to test for diabetes, insulin resistance or hypoglycemia[1]. For this test the patient has ***to fast*** overnight for ***at least*** eight hours. In the morning a drink ***containing*** glucose is given ***orally***. This leads to an increase[2] of the ***blood glucose concentration***. As a consequence insulin secretion is stimulated. ***Within*** two hours the blood glucose level should decrease[3] to normal. A patient with a ***reduced*** insulin secretion or insulin resistance shows a higher blood sugar level than normal after 120 minutes. The test is done in the morning between 8 and 9 a.m. To get a correct test result, the patient has to follow these instructions:

1. Three days before the test, the patient has to eat more than 150 g of ***carbohydrates*** a day.
2. The test cannot be done if the patient has a fever.
3. ***Female patients*** have to do the test at least three days before or after menstruation.

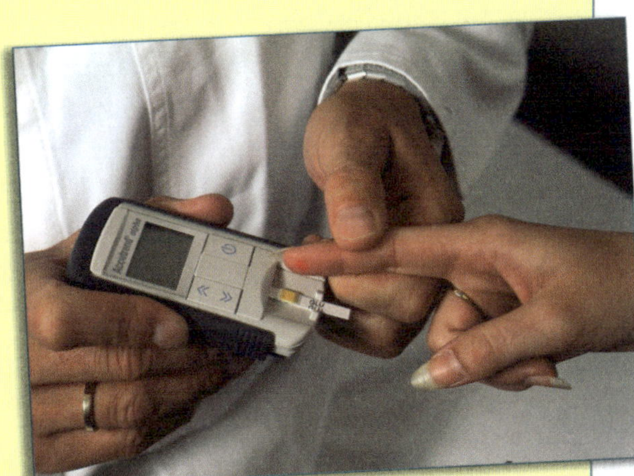

Procedure:

- The fasting blood glucose[4] level is taken.
- Afterwards the patient is given a glucose solution[5] to drink. (1.75 grams of glucose per kg/***bodyweight***, to a maximum dose of 75 g.)
- It should be drunk within 5 minutes.
- A ***blood sample*** is taken after 120 minutes.

When you drink the glucose solution you could get an insulin shock. Therefore the patient ***is not allowed to*** leave the doctor's practice.

Normal Glucose Value		Impaired Glucose Tolerance[6]		Diabetes mellitus	
Fasting	**2hrs**	**Fasting**	**2hrs**	**Fasting**	**2hrs**
< 110 mg/dl	< 140 mg/dl	110 –125 mg/dl	140 – 199 mg/dl	> 125 mg/dl	> 199 mg/dl

Oral Glucose Tolerance Test, diabetes, hypoglycemia, glucose, carbohydrates, menstruation

1 hypoglycemia – low blood sugar level
2 increase – Anstieg
3 to decrease – abfallen, sinken
4 fasting blood glucose or fasting blood sugar – Nüchtern-Blutzucker
5 solution – Lösung
6 impaired glucose tolerance – verminderte Glukosetoleranz

COMPREHENSION

3 **Answer the questions:**

1. Why is the test performed?

 ....

2. How does the patient have to prepare for the test?

 ....

3. When is the test done?

 ....

4. How many blood samples are taken? When are they taken?

 ....

 ....

5. What is the normal fasting glucose level?

 ....

6. Which OGTT result indicates diabetes mellitus?

 ....

 ....

4 **Fill in the gaps with the words below:**

blood glucose level – carbohydrates – diabetes mellitus – diabetes – fast – glucose solution – insulin – insulin shock – normal – oral glucose tolerance test – practice – takes blood – two hours

1. The OGTT .... helps to diagnose ....
2. The day before the test the patient should eat a lot of ....
3. The night before the test he has to ....
4. The next morning the medical assistant .... to find out the ....
5. Then the patient has to drink a .... This stimulates the pancreas to secrete ....
6. After .... another blood sample is taken.
7. During this time he has to stay in the .... because there is a risk of ....
8. A blood glucose level of 110 mg/dl is ....
9. A blood glucose level of 200 mg/dl means that the patient has ....

OGTT-CROSSWORD

5 **Find the correct word for the explanations and write them into the green spaces:**

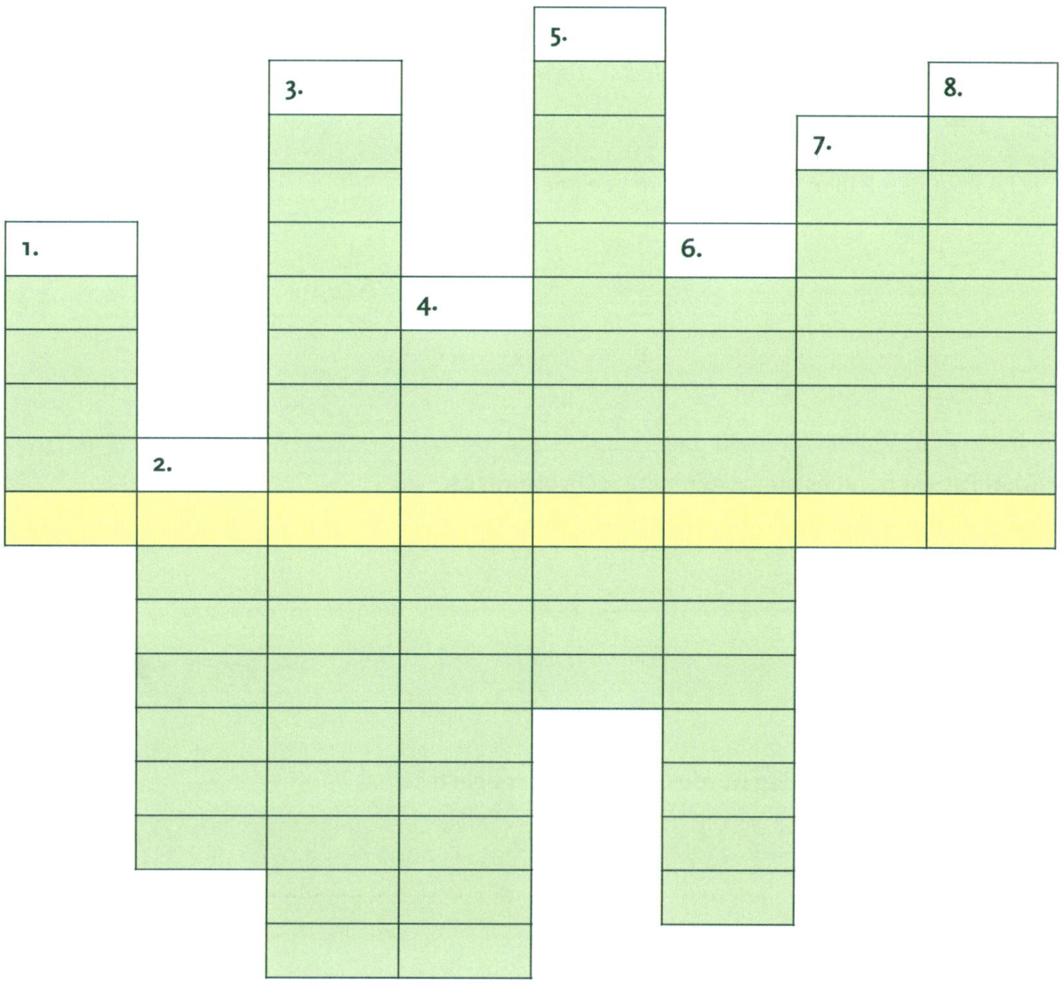

1. an important red fluid in our body
2. it is produced in the pancreas and regulates the blood sugar level
3. a person who assists the doctor
4. a natural energy provider contained in e.g. bread
5. medical term for a low blood sugar level
6. women have it once a month
7. a type of sugar that gives you energy
8. latin word for “honeysweet”

DIALOG / ROLEPLAY

6 **Write a dialog with a partner. Complete the speech bubbles:**

Mr. Mouse is coming out of the consulting room. He needs an appointment for an oral glucose tolerance test because the doctor suspects diabetes mellitus.

MFA fragt den Patienten nach einem geeigneten Termin.

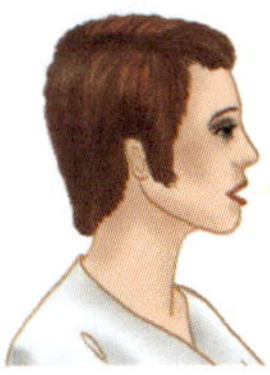

....

....

Dem Patient passt es am besten mittwochvormittags.

....

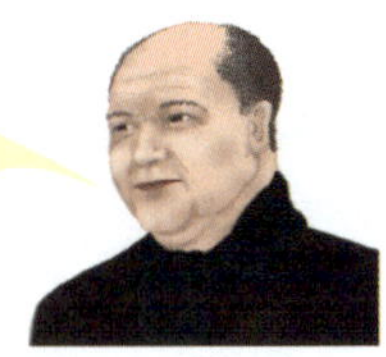

Ein Termin an diesem Tag würde um 8:00 Uhr möglich sein.

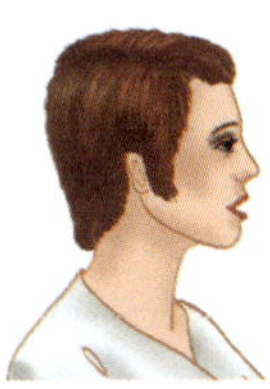

....

Der Patient fragt nach, was ein Glucose-Toleranz-Test eigentlich ist.

....

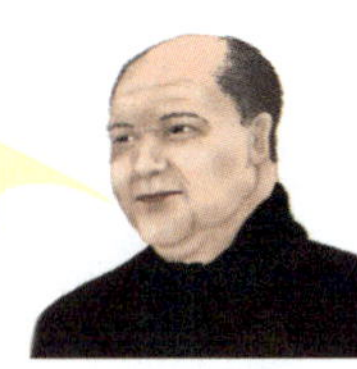

MFA erklärt dem Patienten den Test und die Durchführung.

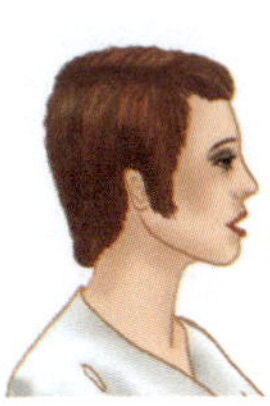

....

....

....

....

....

....

....

Der Patient fragt, ob er vorher irgendetwas beachten muss.

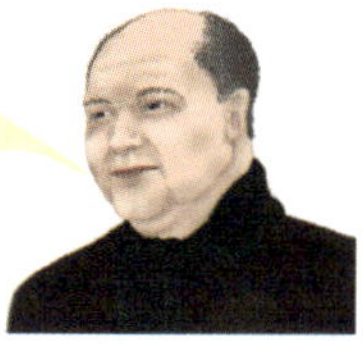

MFA klärt ihn über die Vorbereitung auf.

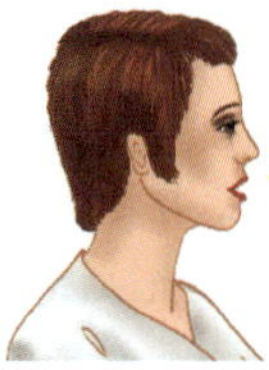

Der Patient möchte wissen, ob er die ganze Zeit über in der Praxis bleiben muss oder ob er zwischenzeitlich auch einkaufen gehen kann.

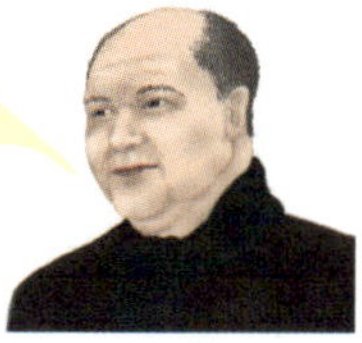

MFA macht ihm deutlich, was für Risiken beim Verlassen der Praxis bestehen.

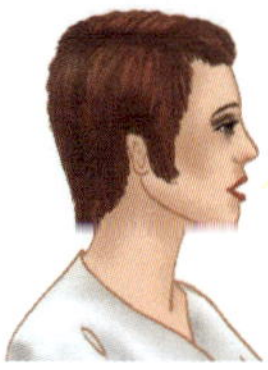

Der Patient bedankt sich fürs erste für die Informationen und verabschiedet sich.

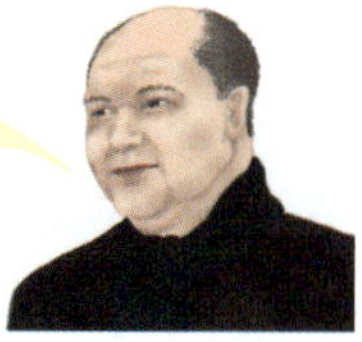

MFA bietet ihm an, dass er bei eventuellen Fragen immer anrufen kann und verabschiedet sich ebenfalls.

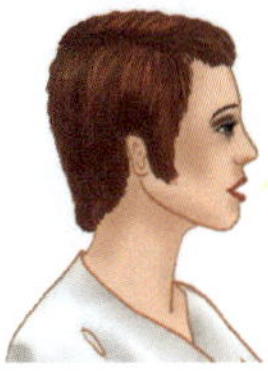

Monitoring the Blood Glucose Level at Home

VOCABULARY

7 **Label the picture with the words in bold from the text above:**

diabetes, glucose, glucometer, lancet, tissue

7 glucometer – Glukosemessgerät
8 to insert – einführen
9 skin puncture – Punktion der Haut
10 lancing device – Stechhilfe
11 site – Stelle
12 index finger – Zeigefinger
13 tissue fluid – Gewebsflüssigkeit
14 to obtain – erhalten, gewinnen

Some patients that have been diagnosed with diabetes have to measure their blood glucose regularly at home. A drop of blood from a finger prick is placed on a ***glucose test strip*** and can then be measured quickly by a small ***glucometer***[7].
First the glucometer has to be prepared by inserting[8] a test strip. To perform a skin puncture[9] the patient can use a sterile ***lancet*** or a ***lancing device***[10]. The finger should be disinfected before puncture. Main puncture sites[11] are the middle finger, ring finger or small ***finger***. The thumb or index finger[12] should not be pricked because you use them for a lot of everyday activities. The site should be punctured quickly and the first drop be wiped away because it contains disinfectant and tissue fluid[13]. Then a drop of blood can be obtained[14] with gentle pressure on either ***puncture site*** and directly be placed on the test strip. The ***glucose level*** can be read after the beep of the glucometer.

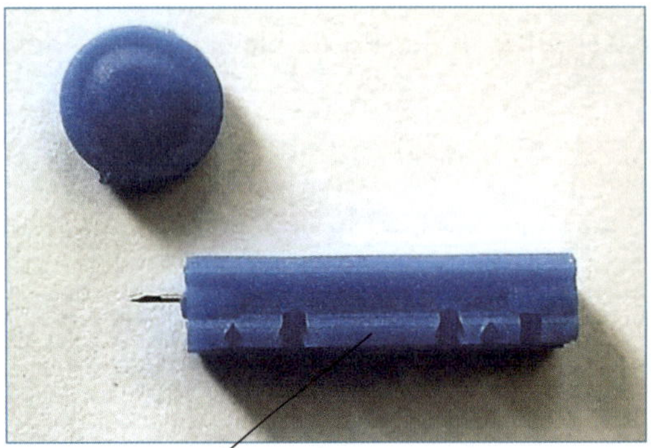

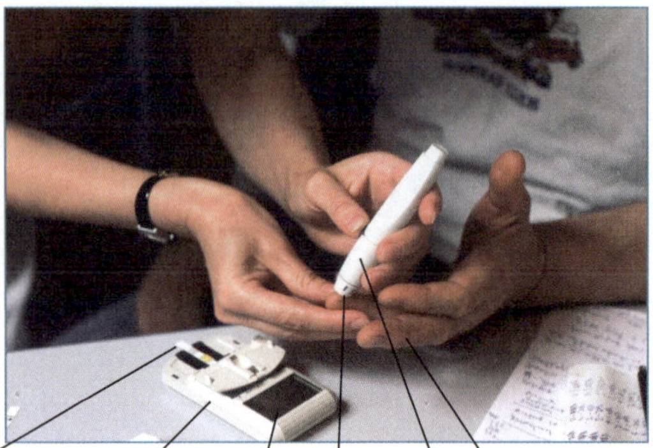

....

....

....

....

....

ROLEPLAY / GIVING INSTRUCTIONS

Mr. Mouse has been diagnosed with diabetes. The doctor wants him to check his blood glucose regularly at home. You have to give him instructions on how to use a glucometer (from your school or practice).

8 **Prepare yourself by writing these instructions down.**

9 **Roleplay a situation where you give instructions to Mr. Mouse.**

18 Wound Management and Tetanus Immunization

LISTENING Track 18

1 **Listen to the dialog and answer the following questions:**

- *What has happened to the patient?*
- *What is the medical assistant doing?*

READING

2 **Read the text and check any new vocabulary in the word list or in a dictionary:**

When the wound bleeds very much a pressure bandage should be applied[1]. It is made of multiple layers[2] of ***gauze*** pads tightly fastened to the skin with tape or bound[3] with ***roller bandage***. Always wait for instructions from the doctor before removing the pressure dressing. The medical assistant is responsible[4] for preparing the ***suture kit***[5] or any other materials to close the wound such as staples[6]. She should ask the patient or a relative what caused the wound and how large and deep it is. It is also important to know when the patient had the last tetanus immunization booster[7]. The doctor will give the order for the necessary immunization(s).

When the bleeding is not severe[8] and there are no foreign bodies, the wound can be cleaned from dirt with ***saline solution***[9]. Don't put alcohol into the wound. Apply antiseptic ointment if the doctor told you to do so. This kills germs and therefore reduces the risk of infection. After the doctor has treated the wound it is the medical assistant's responsibility to apply the dressing. Place a non-sticking pad over the wound. Secure the pad with a ***gauze bandage***. The bandage shouldn't be too tight. Ask the patient if it feels comfortable and check his/her blood circulation. Ask him/her to come back later if it feels too tight. If the injury is over an area that will move, such as the elbow or knee, apply the gauze while the joint is flexed[10] half-way (about 45 degrees). Secure the gauze bandage with a ***self-adhering***[11] ***elastic bandage***. Cut with ***bandage scissors***. Sometimes a wound can also be closed with adhesive[12] ***steri strips***. Usually the patient will be asked to consult the doctor after a few days to check the healing progress and for any signs of infection as well as the removal[13] of the sutures.

gauze,
suture,
immunization,
saline solution,
self-adhering

1 to apply – hier: anlegen
2 layers – Lagen
3 bound – gebunden
4 to be responsible – verantwortlich sein
5 suture kit – Nahtmateriel
6 staples – Klammern
7 tetanus immunization booster – Tetanus Auffrischungsimpfung
8 severe – schwerwiegend
9 saline solution – Kochsalzlösung
10 flexed – gebeugt
11 self-adhering – selbsthaftend
12 adhesive – haftend, klebend
13 removal – Entfernung

VOCABULARY

3 **Match the pictures with the words in bold print in the text above:**

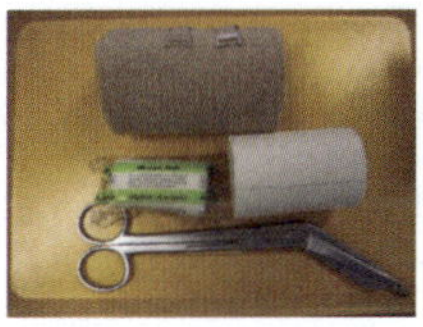	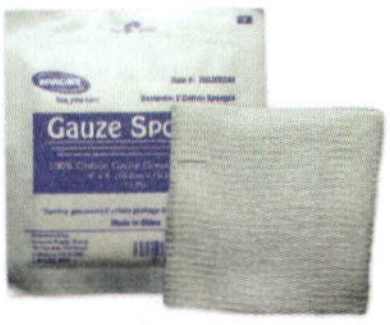	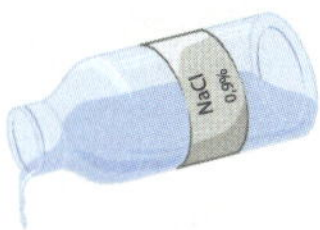	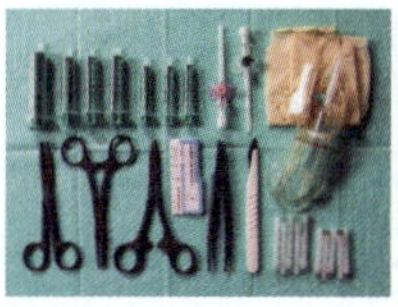	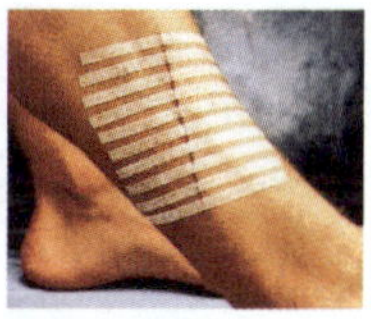

COMPREHENSION

4 **Match the sentence parts correctly:**

14 abrasion – Schürfwunde

1. You have to put pressure on a wound	a. the patient will feel a burning pain.
2. Superficial wounds like abrasions[14]	b. to reduce the risk of infection.
3. After cleaning the wound	c. for his last tetanus immunization booster.
4. Sutures and staples are methods	d. to stop severe bleeding.
5. Gauze bandages are used	e. because there is the risk of poor blood circulation.
6. Sometimes an antiseptic ointment is applied	f. ask him to flex it at a 45 degree angle.
7. Be careful that the bandage is not too tight	g. of closing deep large wounds.
8. Alcohol should not be used because	h. a gauze pad is placed over the wound.
9. If the patient has an injury around his knee	i. first have to be cleaned thoroughly with saline.
10. The medical assistant should ask the patient	j. to fasten a dressing.

5 **What do you say? Write your sentences down in direct speech:**

Fragen Sie die Patientin...

- nach der Ursache für die Wunde.

....

- ob der Verband bequem oder zu fest ist.

....

- wann die Patientin das letzte Mal eine Tetanusimpfung bekommen hat.

....

Sagen Sie der Patientin...

- dass sie ihre Schuhe ausziehen und sich auf die Untersuchungsliege legen soll.

....

- dass Sie jetzt die Wunde säubern.

....

- dass Sie Kompressen mit Salbe auf die Wunde tun und diese dann verbinden.

....

....

- dass sie wiederkommen soll, falls der Verband zu eng ist.

....

- dass sie nach x Tagen sich wieder beim Arzt vorstellen soll.

....

- dass sie nach x Tagen zum Fädenziehen kommen soll.

....

Tetanus Immunization

READING

6 **Read the text and check any new vocabulary in a dictionary:**

What is tetanus?

Tetanus is an infection caused[15] by a bacterium which can cause severe[16] muscles spasms. It affects your nerves and can even be fatal[17]. Tetanus bacteria (germs) live in the soil and dirt. They may get into your body through a wound in the skin. The bacteria produce a toxin (poison) which causes the symptoms. Because it is difficult to treat people should be immunized.

Which effect does the vaccine have?

The vaccine stimulates your body to produce antibodies against the tetanus toxin. These antibodies have a long term effect[18] protecting you from illness should you become infected with this bacterium.

Who should get this vaccine?

All children and adults should be immunized against tetanus. See your doctor if you think that you are not fully immunized. Children are routinely immunized. The tetanus vaccine is normally part of the combined DTP-Polio-Hib vaccine (diphtheria/tetanus/pertussis/polio/ haemophilus influenza b vaccine). Adults and teenagers should be given a combined tetanus/diphtheria/polio vaccine (Td-Polio) as a routine booster[19] every 10 years. Adults who are unsure whether or not they have been fully immunized should catch up with injections. It is important to keep an up-to-date record of all immunizations so that repeat doses do not become necessary.

Do I need a dose of tetanus vaccine after cuts, bites, etc?

If you are not immunized or up-to-date with boosters then an injection of vaccine is usually given. If your wound is very dirty then an injection of human tetanus antiserum which contains antibodies is usually given (passive immunization), no matter whether you have been immunized against tetanus or not. It has an immediate[20] effect and gives extra protection against tetanus.

How is this vaccine given?

After disinfecting the injection site it is given in the anterolateral[21] thigh muscle (for infants and young toddlers) or in the deltoid muscle (for older children and adults). If passive and active vaccines are given simultaneously, the vaccines are injected into different sites, for example the left and right arm. Otherwise there is the risk that the vaccines will neutralize each other and have no effect. This could be the case if the patient has not received a booster for more than 10 years. If the patient receives anticoagulation treatment (e.g. Marcumar®) the vaccine has to be injected subcutaneously to avoid the risk of intramuscular bleeding.

Are there any side-effects from the tetanus vaccine?

Some people get a slight redness and swelling around the injection site[22] which disappears after a few days. You might feel slightly unwell for a day with a mild headache, tiredness, slight muscle aches or a mild fever. Severe reactions are extremely rare.

Who should not receive the tetanus vaccine?

If you have a fever, you should wait with the injection until the illness has gone (unless the dose is needed because of a wound). You should also not get another vaccination if a previous injection caused a severe reaction. The tetanus vaccine is safe if you are pregnant or breastfeeding.

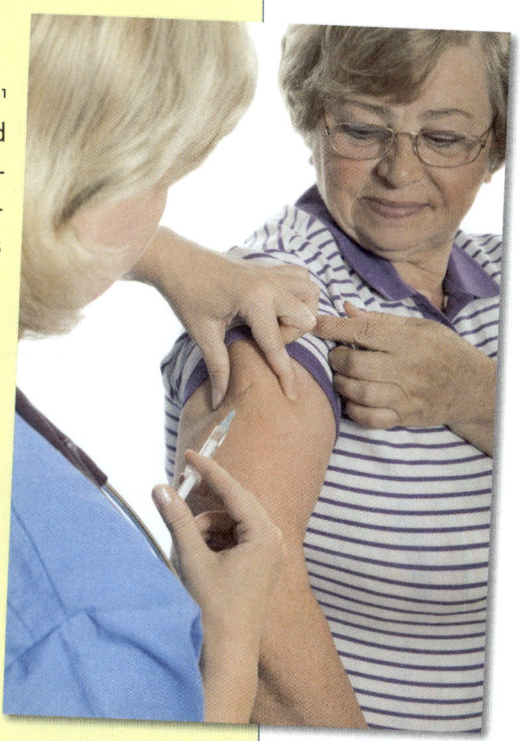

immunization, muscles, immunize, vaccine, diphtheria, haemophilus influenza, antiserum, anterolateral, deltoid, anticoagulation, subcutaneous, intramuscular

15 to cause – verursachen
16 severe – schwerwiegend
17 fatal – fatal, tödlich
18 long term effect – Langzeitwirkung
19 booster – Auffrischungsimpfung
20 immediate – sofortig
21 antero – vordere/r/s
lateral – äußere/r/s
22 site – Stelle

COMPREHENSION

7 **Match the words with their definition:**

1. fatal	a small injection that you are given some time after a larger injection to keep the protection effective
2. wound	b. injecting antibodies
3. toxin	c. injured skin
4. active immunization	d. get
5. passive immunization	e. young child that has just learned to walk
6. booster	f. injecting dead or harmless agents
7. receive	g. under the skin
8. simultaneously	h. deadly
9. infant	i. at the same time
10. toddler	j. poison
11. subcutaneous	k. baby
12. disinfect	l. reduce germs

8 **Correct these false statements:**

1. Tetanus is a viral infection causing muscle relaxation through toxins.

   ....

2. You cannot catch tetanus if you cut yourself during garden work.

   ....

3. Because you cannot protect yourself against this infection you should have no animal contact.

   ....

4. As an adult you need further tetanus boosters every 5 years to be protected.

   ....

5. A medical assistant never has to ask the patient if he/she is immunized against tetanus.

   ....

   ....

6. The tetanus vaccine is given intramuscularly into the arm or breast muscle.

   ....

7. Patients taking anticoagulants must not get the tetanus vaccine.

   ....

8. A patient with a wound always gets a tetanus antiserum.

   ....

   ....

9. Injecting the antiserum is an active immunization.

   ....

10. You can inject the vaccine and the antiserum into the same injection site.

11. Most people suffer side effects like severe redness or swelling.

12. Anybody can be immunized against tetanus at any time.

DIALOG / ROLEPLAY

9 **Write a dialog with a partner. Complete the speech bubbles:**

Felipe dos Santos, a football player, comes into your practice because he was fouled in the match. He has a dirty bleeding abrasion on his right knee. The doctor asks you to treat the wound.

Part A

At the reception

Der Patient kommt direkt vom Fußballfeld in die Praxis und berichtet, was vorgefallen ist. Er möchte gerne den Arzt sehen, weil sein Knie blutet und schmerzt.

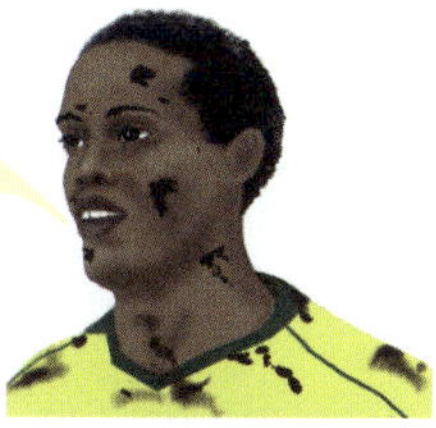

Bevor die MFA nach der Versichertenkarte fragt, begleitet sie den Patienten ins Wartezimmer, damit er sich setzen kann.

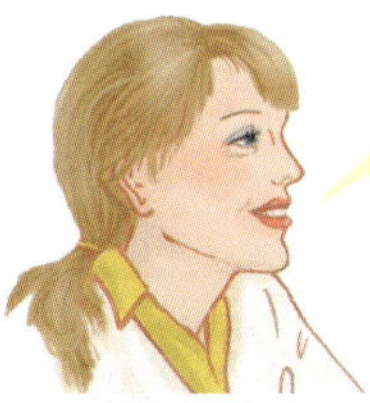

After the consultation

MFA bittet den Patienten ins Verbandszimmer und bittet ihn, die Schuhe auszuziehen und sich auf die Untersuchungsliege zu legen.

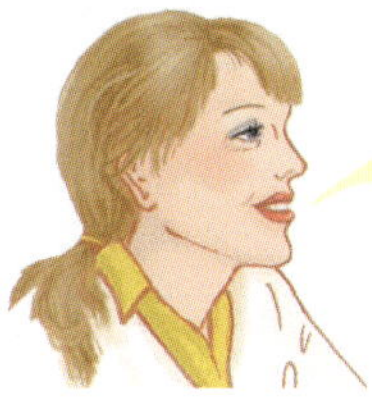

MFA kündigt an, dass sie zunächst die Wunde reinigen wird. Dann schmiert sie etwas Salbe mit einer Kompresse auf die Wunde und fragt den Patienten, ob alles in Ordnung ist.

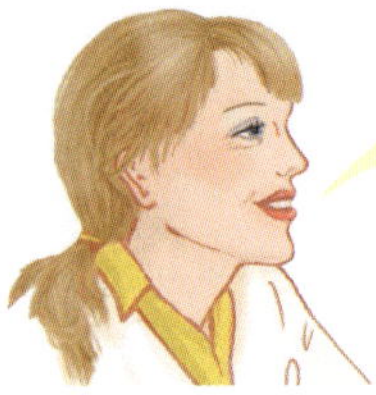

Der Patient sagt, dass es kaum schmerzt. Er fragt, was die Salbe bewirkt.

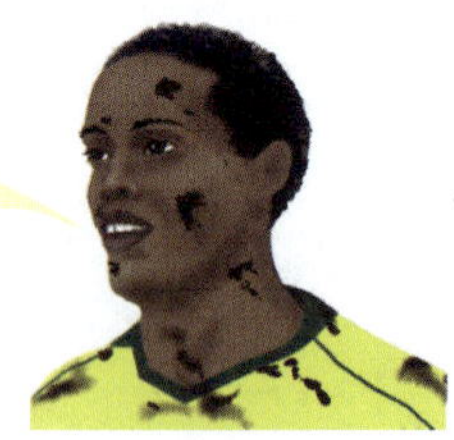

Die Salbe wirkt antiseptisch.
MFA möchte jetzt die Wunde verbinden. Sie fragt den Patienten, ob der Verband zu eng ist.

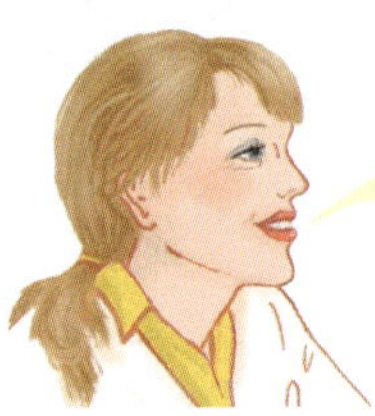

Der Patient findet, dass der Verband perfekt sitzt.

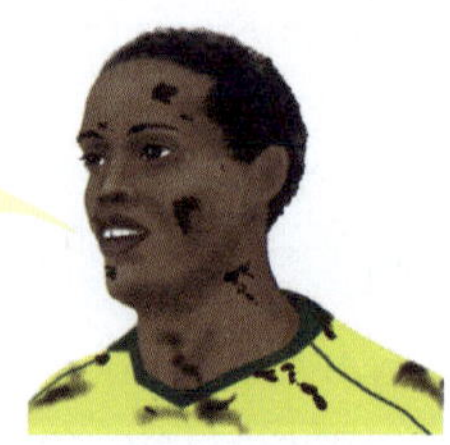

MFA bittet den Patienten, sofort wiederzukommen, falls der Verband doch zu eng sein sollte.

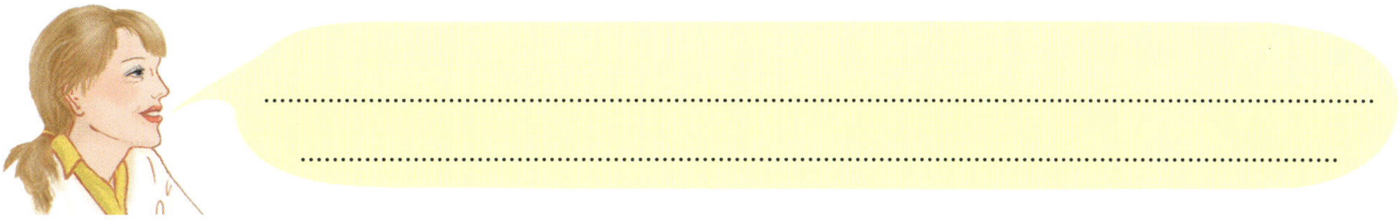

Part B

MFA fragt den Patienten, wann er die letzte Tetanusauffrischung bekam.

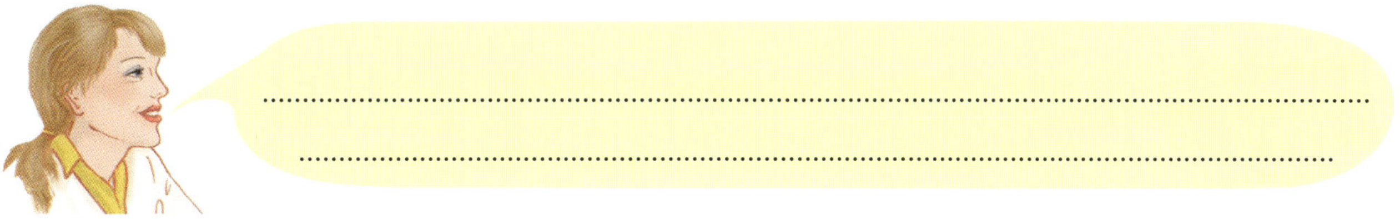

Der Patient ist sich unsicher. Er fragt, warum das wichtig ist.

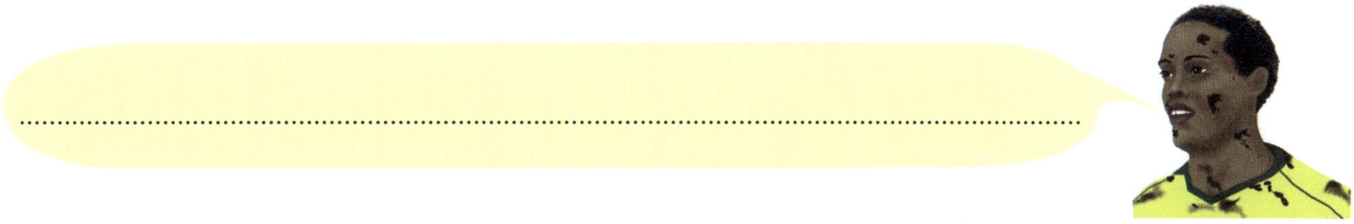

MFA erklärt, dass eine Gefahr besteht, falls nicht mehr genug Impfschutz vorhanden ist, da sehr viel Dreck und Erde in der Wunde ist. Sie fragt, ob er den Impfausweis dabei hat.

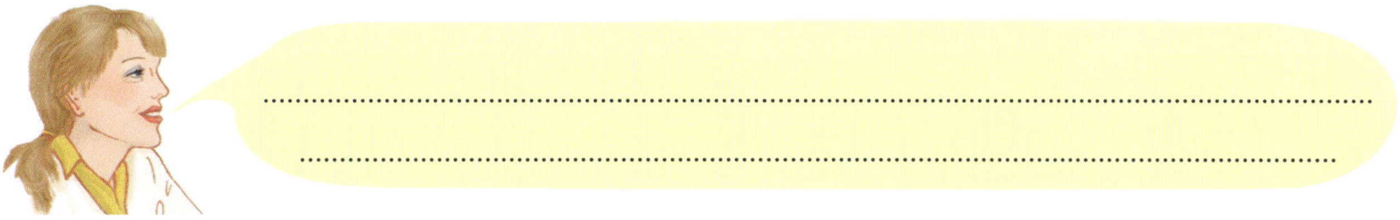

Den Impfausweis hat er nicht dabei.
Der Patient ist sicher, dass es sehr lange her ist.

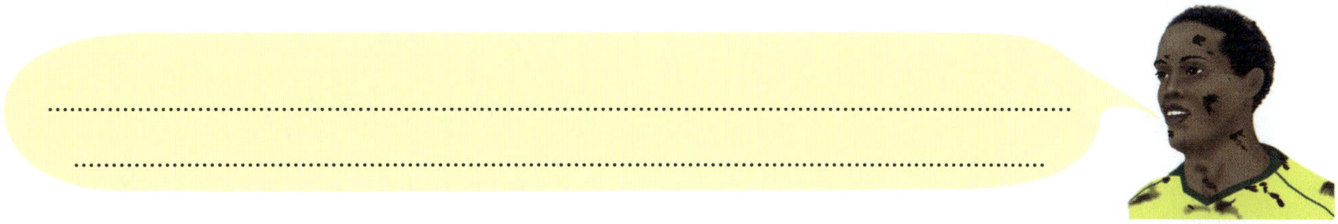

MFA teilt ihm mit, dass er dann zwei Spritzen bekommen wird, damit er auch sicher geschützt ist. Sie erklärt, dass die eine Spritze eine sofortige Wirkung und die andere eine langfristige Wirkung hat.

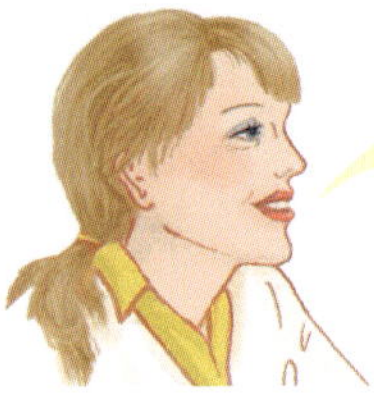

Den Patienten beruhigt das, da ihm bekannt ist, dass Wundstarrkrampf sehr gefährlich ist.

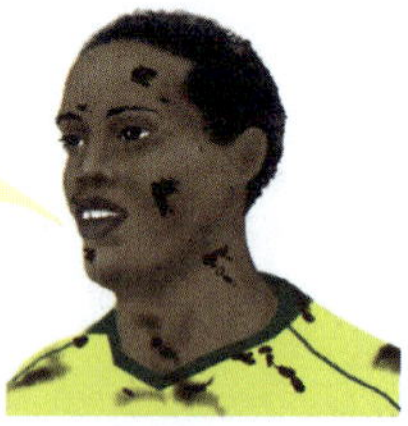

MFA hält Rücksprache mit dem Arzt, nimmt die Impfstoffe aus dem Kühlschrank und teilt dem Patienten mit, dass er die erste Spritze in den rechten Oberarm und die zweite in den linken bekommt. Sie desinfiziert die Einstichstellen und sagt, dass es kalt wird.

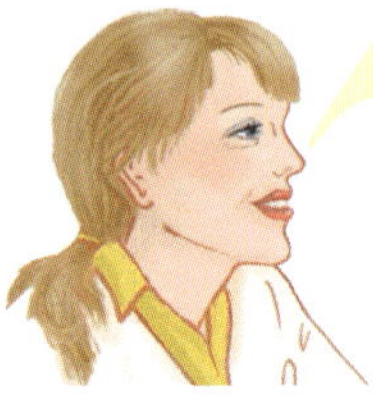

MFA klärt ihn über mögliche Nebenwirkungen auf. Dann injiziert sie die Impfstoffe und versorgt sie mit einem Pflaster.

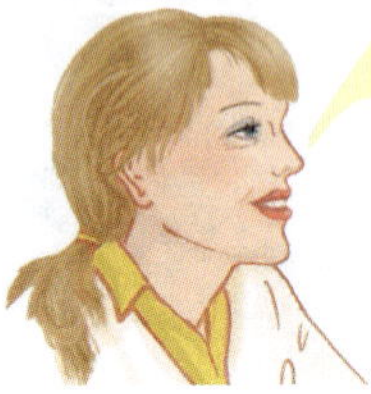

Der Patient äußert, dass es überhaupt nicht weh getan hat.

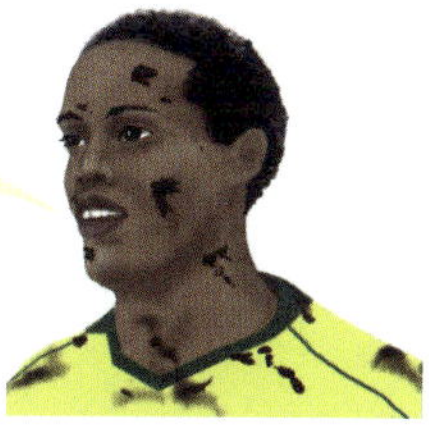

MFA stellt ihm eine Bescheinigung über die Impfung aus und bittet ihn, den Impfausweis zu bringen, damit die Impfung dokumentiert werden kann. Sie bittet ihn, in zwei Tagen zum Verbandswechsel wiederzukommen. Bis dahin soll er nicht duschen oder baden, weil die Wunde nicht mit Wasser in Kontakt kommen darf.

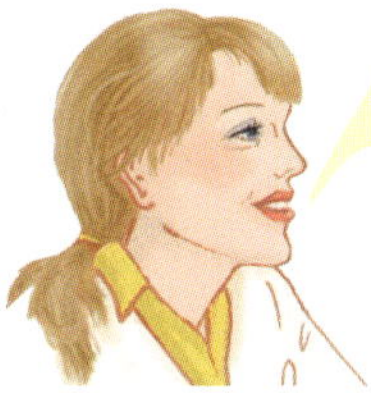

Der Patient bedankt und verabschiedet sich.

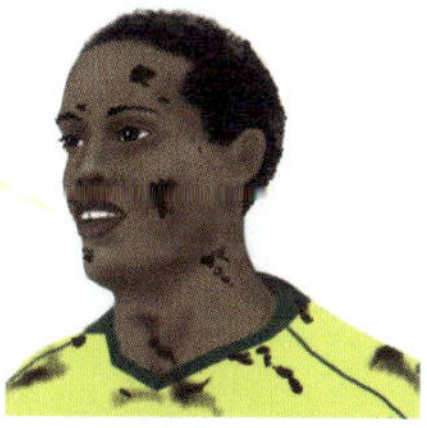

MFA wünscht ihm gute Besserung und verabschiedet sich.

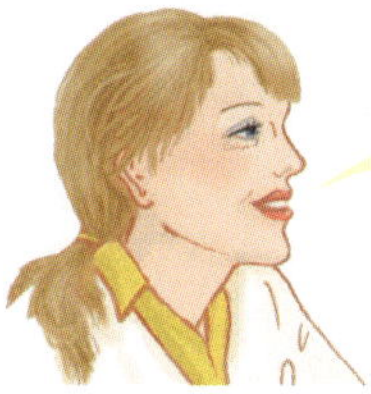

Wound-Tetanus WORD SEARCH

8 **Can you find 37 hidden words? Find the hidden message in the remaining letters:**

G	N	O	I	T	C	E	F	N	I	V	A	C	C	I	N	E	H
E	N	O	I	T	A	L	U	C	R	I	C	D	O	O	L	B	E
E	T	S	A	P	T	S	E	B	A	C	T	E	R	I	U	M	A
T	T	A	M	N	R	E	T	S	O	O	B	E	B	F	E	Y	L
S	O	I	L	S	T	O	U	L	S	B	S	S	L	O	V	R	I
O	E	O	S	P	A	N	T	S	U	P	T	U	E	R	I	U	N
S	A	H	A	N	H	P	A	E	O	D	E	T	E	E	T	J	G
S	T	N	C	N	O	Y	S	N	C	R	A	U	D	I	A	N	P
S	T	E	T	A	T	I	S	E	G	T	E	R	I	G	L	I	R
E	E	H	R	I	E	I	T	I	L	E	I	E	N	N	E	S	O
N	N	L	G	I	B	L	S	C	C	C	R	O	G	B	R	W	G
D	G	I	P	I	S	O	C	E	E	I	S	P	N	O	E	E	R
E	V	E	L	A	T	T	D	S	P	J	A	U	E	D	V	L	E
R	R	I	R	A	T	Y	R	I	U	T	N	N	M	Y	E	L	S
T	T	E	N	M	S	S	Y	I	E	M	I	I	E	A	S	I	S
Y	G	N	I	S	S	E	R	D	P	S	R	C	W	O	U	N	D
S	I	D	E	E	F	F	E	C	T	S	B	A	N	D	A	G	E
T	N	E	M	T	N	I	O	T	C	E	F	N	I	S	I	D	S

Hidden message:

19 Removing Stitches

LISTENING Track 19

1 **Listen to the dialog and answer the following questions:**

- *Why is the patient in the doctor's practice?*
- *What instructions does the medical assistant give?*

READING

2 **Read the text and check any vocabulary in the word list or in a dictionary:**

Procedure

Step one:
Disinfect your hands, put on the gloves, remove the old dressing or band-aid which might be on the stitched wound and disinfect the whole area.

Step two:
Unpack the sterile pair of tweezers. Be careful that all your instruments stay sterile, which means do not touch or cough on them. Disinfect the wound again and unpack the sterile scalpel or sterile blade.

Step three:
Take the sterile pair of tweezers and take one end of the thread from the wound. It is best if you take the knot. Pull a little bit on the thread to see where you have to cut it. You need to make a cut under the knot because if you take the other side, the microorganisms which are on the thread go through the skin. The consequence of this can be an infection and inflammation of the wound.

Step four:
Disinfect the wound again and put a sterile dressing on it. Put the pair of tweezers and pair of scissors in a sterilizing bath and put the rest into the waste bin. Tell the patient that the wound must not come into contact with water for the next three days.

sterile,
cough,
microorganisms

VOCABULARY

3 **Match the words with the pictures:**

sterile pair of tweezers – sterile cotton swab – disinfectant – sterile pair of scissors – band-aid – gloves

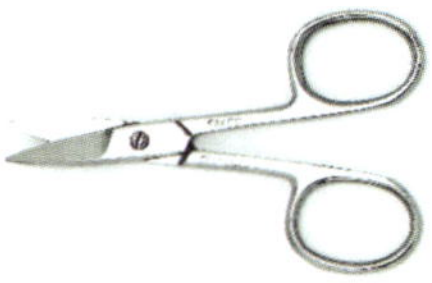
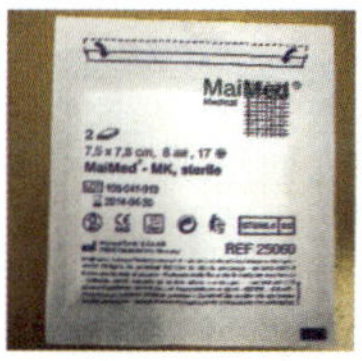
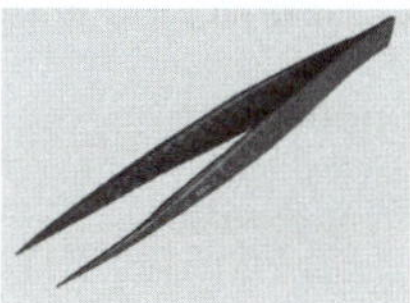
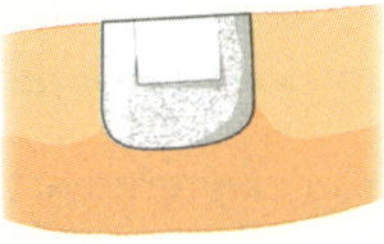
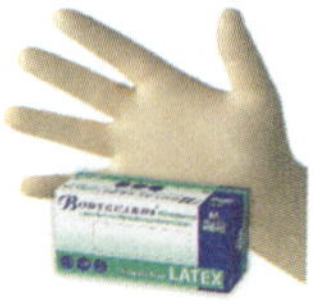
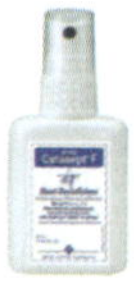

....

....

COMPREHENSION

4 **Answer the questions:**

1. What is important before removing stitches? Hint: It's something to do with your hands.

   ....

2. Do you have to disinfect the wound? If so, why?

   ....

3. Name five materials you need to remove stitches.

   ....

   ....

4. How should you treat the wound after having removed the stitches?

   ....

5. How do you remove the stitches? Is it wise to cut through all the stitches at once? Why/ why not?

   ....

   ....

6. How long does the patient have to keep the wound dry for?

   ....

5 **Fill in the gaps with the words below:**

pair of scissors | thread | sterile dressing | needle | gloves | suture | scar | pair of tweezers | microorganisms | disinfectant | examine

1. You can minimize microorganisms in a wound with a ....
2. You have to wear .... while you remove the stitches.
3. The doctor has to .... the wound before you remove the stitches.
4. A mark left on the skin after healing of injured tissue is called a ....
5. A medical term for a closed wound with a thread is ....
6. To close a wound you need .... and ....
7. You can remove the thread with a ....
8. You need these to cut the thread: ....
9. After having removed the stitches you have to protect the wound with a ....
10. You reduce .... with a disinfectant.

DIALOG / ROLE PLAY

6 **Write a dialog with a partner. Complete the speech bubbles:**

A patient, Lalit Kumar, comes into your practice to have his foot checked because he had an operation ten days ago. The doctor examines the wound and wants you to remove the stitches. You take the material you need and go into the treatment room.

MFA begrüßt den Patienten und erklärt, dass sie die Fäden im Fuß entfernen will. Sie greift zum Desinfektionsmittel und desinfiziert die genähte Stelle.

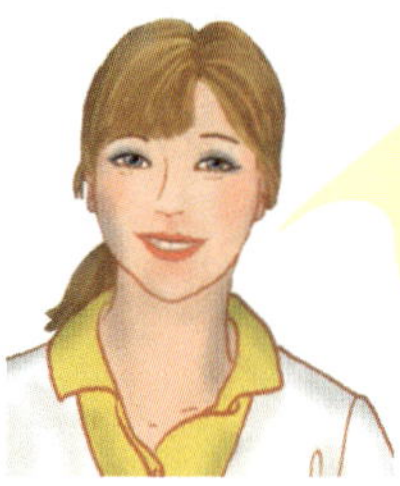

Der Patient äußert, dass er Angst vor Schmerzen hat .

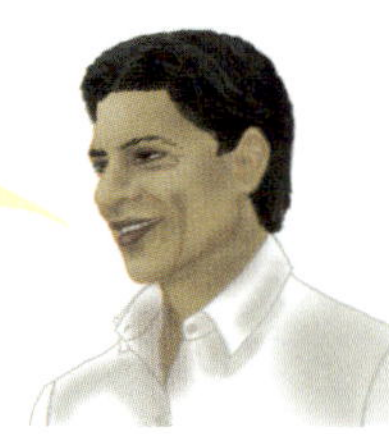

MFA erklärt, dass es nicht schmerzen wird, jedoch wird er ein leichtes Kribbeln merken. Sie fragt den Patienten, ob er bereit ist.

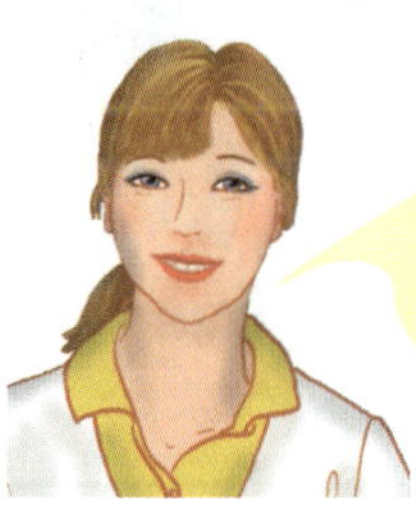

Der Patient ist bereit.

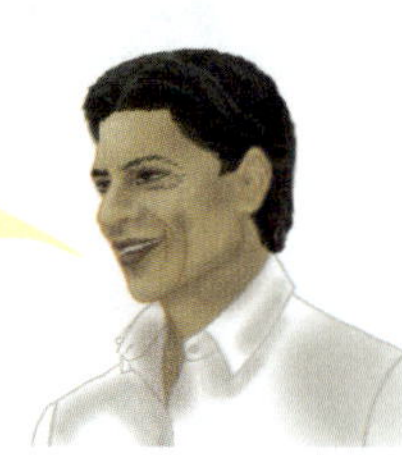

MFA erklärt, dass sie die Wunde erneut desinfiziert und die Fäden mit einer Pinzette entfernen wird.

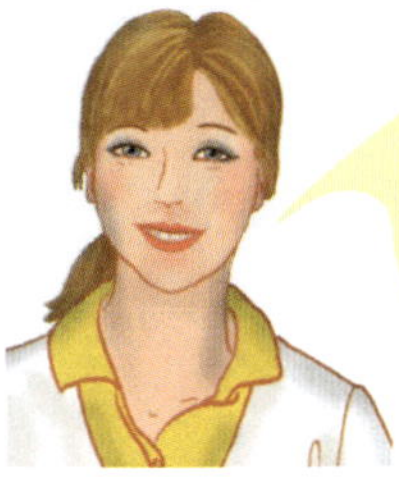

MFA ist fertig und versorgt die Wunde mit einem sterilen Wundschnellverband.
Dann weist sie darauf hin, dass der Patient in den nächsten drei Tagen die Wunde noch nicht waschen soll.

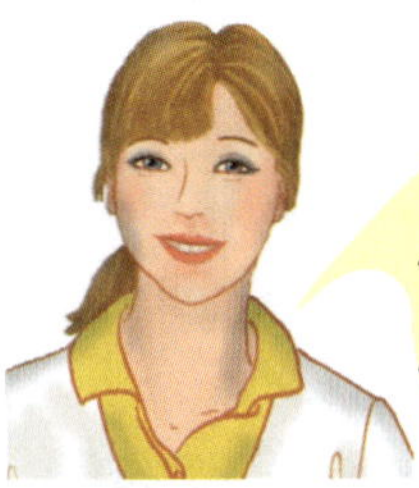

Der Patient lobt die MFA, da es kaum weh getan hat, bedankt sich und wünscht einen schönen Tag.

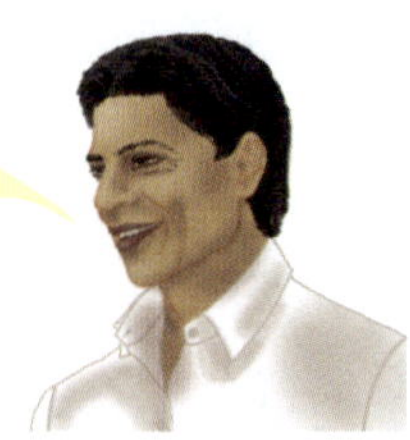

MFA bedankt sich und wünscht ebenfalls einen schönen Tag

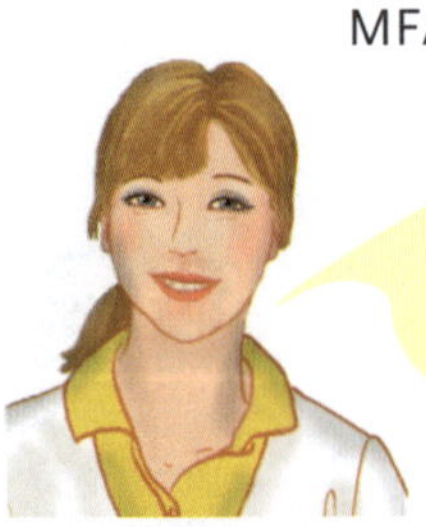

20 Allergy Testing

LISTENING Track 20

1 **Listen to the dialog and answer the following questions:**

- *Why is the patient in the doctor's practice?*
- *What is the medical assistant doing?*

READING

2 **Read the following text and find the German words 3. Check any other new vocabulary in the vocabulary list or in a dictionary.**

Text	
The function of your immune system is to protect you from infections. If you have allergies, it overreacts and fights normally harmless substances like dust mites, animal hair, pollen, foods or latex. Some of these allergens cause sneezing, a runny nose, itchy eyes and ears, and a sore throat. Others, such as foods, may cause wheals (a red, bumpy, itchy skin rash), stomach cramps, vomiting, or diarrhea. Allergens can cause breathing problems like wheezing and shortness of breath (asthma). Some allergens, such as foods, are a problem all year long. If you are allergic to pollen from trees, you will only have problems in spring. The doctor will ask you a lot of questions about your symptoms, the animals and plants in your home, your family history, and about the foods you eat. An allergist may do a skin prick or scratch test. Small liquid drops of the allergens are placed on your forearm, upper arm or back including a positive and a negative control to see whether the test works. Then your skin will be pricked a bit so the allergen goes under the skin's surface. You will feel a quick pinch. You have to wait for about 20 minutes. During that time you must not move or touch your arm and you are not allowed to scratch if you feel any itching. After a short while a wheal (bumpy, itchy and red spot – like a mosquito bite) will develop where the positive control was applied on the skin. It shows that the test has worked. Every further wheal shows an allergic reaction. Before the test you have to stop taking antihistamine medications for several days, because they may lead to falsely negative results. Skin tests may itch for a while. You might get an antihistamine or steroid cream after the test to reduce the itching. The patient always needs to be carefully observed because allergy testing bears the risk of anaphylactic shock. Some doctors may also test your blood for IgE antibodies that signal an allergic reaction. Your doctor sometimes prescribes antiallergic medicine. If your symptoms do not get better by staying away from allergens and taking medicines, an allergist might recommend allergy injections. These injections should make your immune system less sensitive to the allergen.	

immune system, wheals, stomach, diarrhea, allergen, asthma, antihistamine, steroid, anaphylactic shock

COMPREHENSION

3 **Find the following words in the text:**

Immunsystem | vor Infektionen schützen | harmlos

Hausstaubmilben | Nahrungsmittel | Niesen | Augenjucken

Halsschmerzen | Quaddeln | Erbrechen | Durchfall | Pfeifen

Kurzatmigkeit | Frühjahr | Beschwerden | Allergologe

flüssig | Unterarm | (ein-)stechen, „pieksen“ | Zwicken

Ritz, Kratzer | allergisch sein | falsch negativ | jucken

eine Zeitlang | genau beobachten | ein Risiko tragen | Antikörper

empfehlen | Spritze, Injektion | weniger empfindlich | verschreiben

Allergene meiden

4 **Structure the text (2). Match the headings below with sections of the text. Write the number of headings next to the text:**

definition of the term “allergy”

allergy diagnosis

allergy therapy

allergy symptoms

prick test procedure

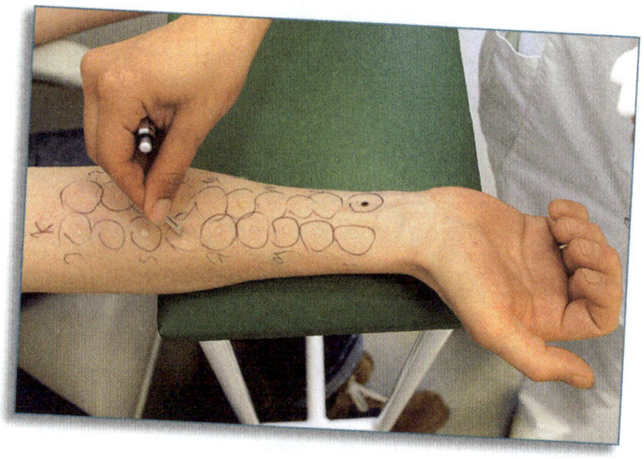

5 **Correct these false statements:**

1. When you have an allergy your immune system fights pathologic germs.

....

....

2. Food allergens mostly cause itchy eyes and sneezing.

....

....

3. Many people are allergic to animal hair in spring.

....

4. A stool test is done to diagnose an allergy.

....

5. A prick test is usually done on your leg or upper arm.

....

6. The patient will not feel anything when the skin is pricked or scratched.

....

7. If the patient is allergic to one of the allergens placed on his/her skin, the skin will show a bumpy, itchy and white mosquito bite.

....

....

8. Before the test, the patient mustn't take paracetamol.

....

9. After the test the patient might get an antihistamine cream to relieve the burn.

....

10. Sometimes a urine sample has to be taken to check for antibodies.

....

11. Sometimes the patient gets a prescription for painkillers to treat the allergy.

....

12. Allergy injections should make the immune system allergic to the allergen.

....

DIALOG / ROLEPLAY

6 **Write a dialog with a partner:**

Mrs. Murray has been suffering from indigestion with abdominal cramps for a while. Her GP wants to rule out an allergy and referred her to the allergist Dr. Watson for a skin prick test.

MFA begrüßt die Patientin.

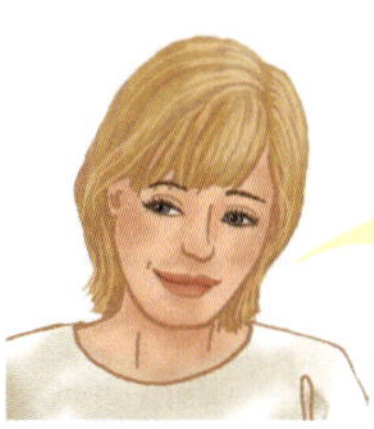

....

Die Patientin stellt sich vor, sie hat einen Termin zum Allergietest um 15:30 Uhr.

....

....

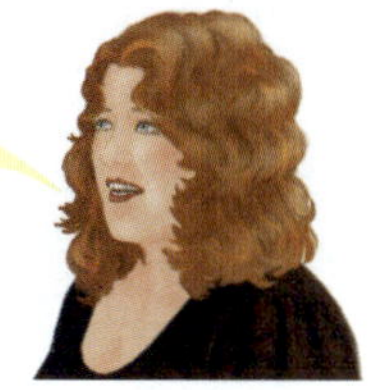

MFA bittet um KVK und bittet die Patientin, ihr ins Behandlungszimmer zu folgen und auf dem blauen Stuhl Platz zu nehmen.

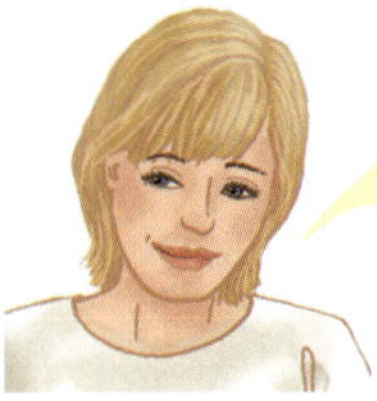

Die Patientin gibt MFA die KVK, folgt ihr ins Behandlungszimmer und setzt sich.

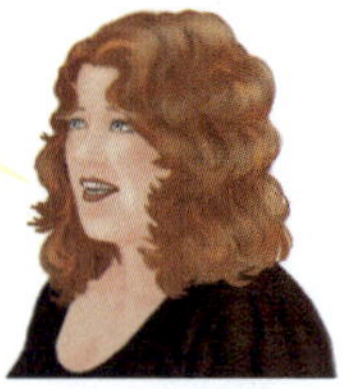

MFA teilt mit, dass sie die Haut auf dem Unterarm desinfiziert und dann mit einem Stift die Teststellen kennzeichnet. Anschließend trägt sie jeweils einen Tropfen der Allergieextrakte auf. MFA teilt der Patientin mit, dass sie jetzt die Allergieextrakte mit einer Lanzette in die Haut einritzen muss.

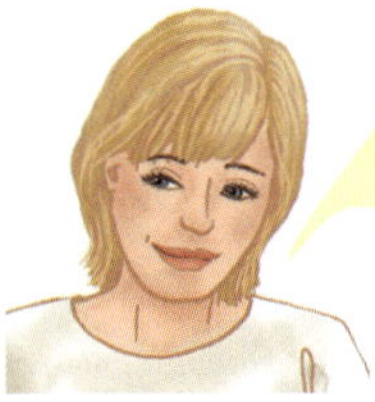

Die Patientin fragt, ob es schmerzhaft ist.

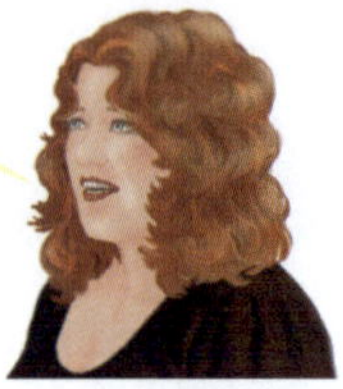

MFA erklärt, dass die Patientin nur ein kurzes Zwicken merken wird. Nach kurzer Zeit wird sich eine Quaddel bilden, die wie ein Mückenstich aussieht und anzeigt, dass der Test funktioniert. Jede weitere Quaddel zeigt eine allergische Reaktion an. MFA fordert die Patientin auf, ruhig sitzen zu bleiben, den Arm nicht zu berühren und bei Juckreiz nicht zu kratzen.

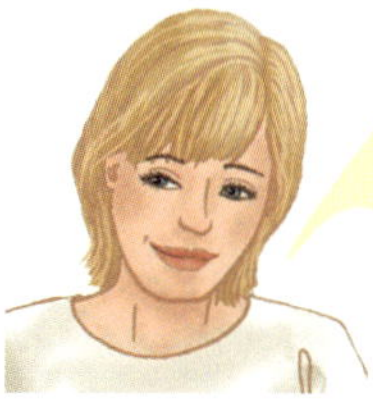

Die Patientin fragt, wie lange der Test dauert.

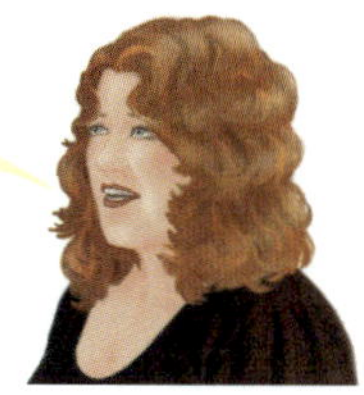

MFA teilt mit, dass die Patientin nun ca. 20 Minuten warten muss.

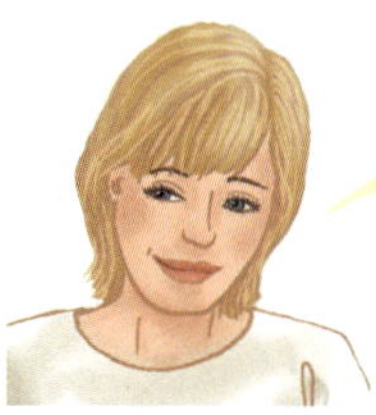

after 20 minutes

MFA erklärt, dass sich bei der Testkontrolle eine Quaddel gebildet hat, so wie sie zuvor erklärte. Bei den anderen Punkten ist keine Reaktion zu erkennen und man kann davon ausgehen, dass keine Allergien gegen die Testsubstanzen bestehen. MFA teilt der Patientin mit, dass der Arzt noch einen Blick darauf werfen wird und sie sich noch kurz gedulden muss.

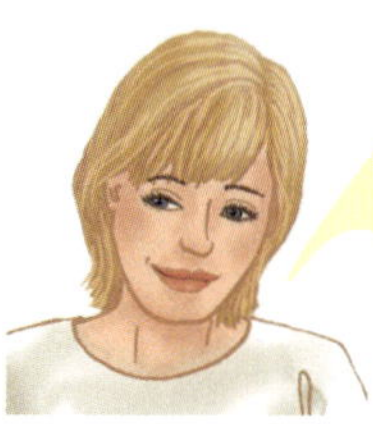

Die Patientin ist erleichtert und teilt mit, dass das eine gute Nachricht ist.

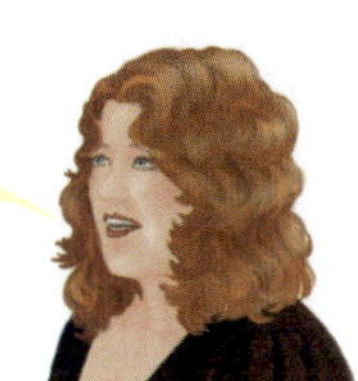

Nach der Begutachtung des Arztes säubert die MFA den Arm der Patientin mit Alkohol. Nachdem sie fertig ist, verabschiedet sie sich freundlich.

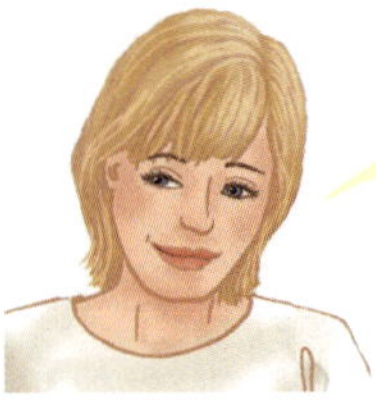

Die Patientin bedankt und verabschiedet sich.

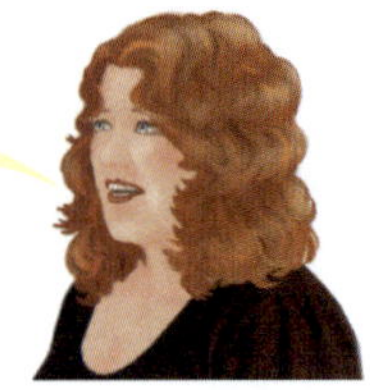

Allergy Test WORD SEARCH

7 **Can you find 24 hidden words? Find the hidden message in the remaining letters:**

A H M E T S Y S E N U M M I S
P N T G P I N C H R E A H S O
F R T A N O H A I Y S L S E R
F O I I E I L A E V O L A T E
E R R C A R H L I S N E R I T
S A G E K L B C E C Y R N M H
O S M N A T L F T N N G I T R
H M E M I R E E O I N E K S O
C O I L N Z M S R T U N S U A
T N A L M L E E T G R D R D T
A D I A R R H E A G I O O Y M
R A M H T S A X N D A C H O Y
C G N I Z E E H W S D R S S F
S T O M A C H C R A M P S A R
S E N S I T I V E S L A E H W

Hidden message:

21 Audiometry / Hearing test

LISTENING Track 21

1 **Listen to the dialog and answer the following questions:**

- *Why is the patient in the doctor's practice?*
- *What is the medical assistant doing?*

READING

2 **Read the following text and find the German words 3. Check any other new vocabulary in the vocabulary list or in a dictionary.**

audiometry, audiogram, decibels, surgery

Audiometry tests a person's ability to hear various sound frequencies. By doing an audometric test, a doctor (e.g. an ENT[1] specialist) can diagnose hearing problems like hardness of hearing or even hearing loss resulting in deafness.

The most popular method is sound-audiometry which has to be performed in a sound-proof testing room. The patient wears a set of headphones which block out other distracting sounds and send a test tone to one ear at a time. The patient is asked to press a button or raise a hand to indicate that he/she has heard something. Then the volume is lowered until the patient can no longer detect the sound. This process is repeated over a wide range of tones from very deep to very high sounds. Each ear is tested separately.

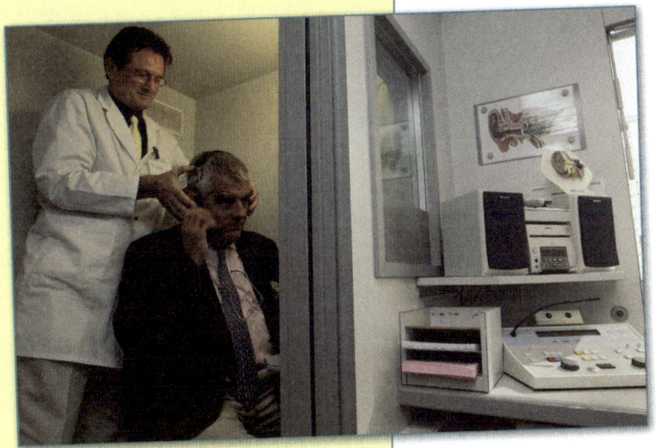

A second test uses a headband with small rectangles which are placed behind the ears to conduct sound through the bones of the skull. The vibrations are transmitted to the inner ear. The tones are also repeated at various volumes and frequencies.

The results are recorded in an audiogram and show the hearing potential of the person. Hearing is measured in decibels. An adult with normal hearing can detect sounds between 0 – 20 decibels. If a hearing impairment is diagnosed the doctor can prescribe hearing aids, surgery or speech therapy.

1 ENT specialist (ear, nose and throat doctor) – HNO Doktor

COMPREHENSION

3 **Find the following words in the text:**

Fähigkeit · verschiedene · Klangfrequenzen · Arzt
Schwerhörigkeit · Hörverlust/Taubheit · schallisoliert · Kopfhörer
Störgeräusche · liefern · zur Zeit · anzeigen
Lautstärke verringern · wahrnehmen · Bandbreite · getrennt
Stirnband · Rechteck · leiten · Schädel · Hörgerät
Hörbeeinträchtigung · Operation · Sprachtherapie

4 **Answer the following questions:**

1. What can be diagnosed with an audiography?

   ....

   ....

2. What is needed to perform an audiometric test?

   ....

3. What kind of sounds are played to the patient?

   ....

4. How does the test person indicate that he/she has heard something?

   ....

5. Are both ears tested at the same time?

   ....

6. What is the difference between the first and the second test?

   ....

   ....

7. What unit of measurement is used to describe hearing?

   ....

8. Name a possible therapy if a person suffers from hearing impairment.

   ....

DIALOG / ROLEPLAY

5 **Write a dialog with a partner. Complete the speech bubbles:**

Mrs. Shell is a little worried that her left ear could be damaged because she has had otitis media on that side of the ear three times in her life. She feels she can hear better with her right ear. Last week she made an appointment with an ENT specialist. Today is the appointment for an audiometric test.

MFA begrüßt die Patientin.

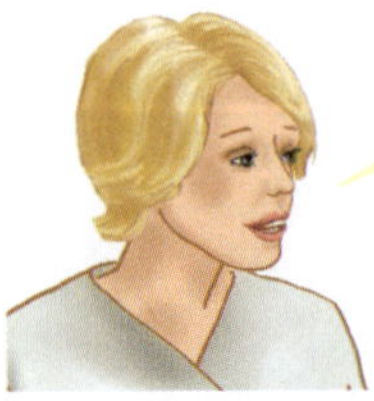

....

Die Patientin stellt sich vor und sagt, dass sie einen Termin zum Hörtest hat.

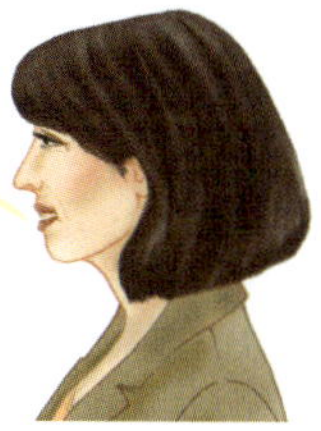

MFA fragt die Patientin nach ihrer Versichertenkarte.

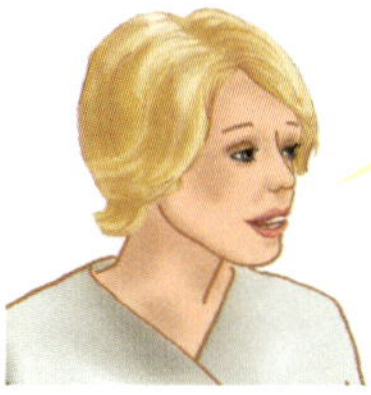

Die Patientin antwortet und überreicht die KVK.

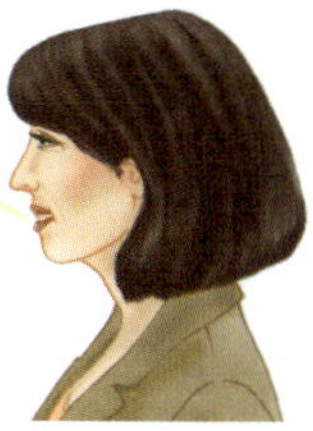

MFA liest die KVK ein und gibt sie zurück.
Sie fordert die Patientin auf, im Wartezimmer Platz zu nehmen. Sie teilt der Patientin mit, dass sie in ein paar Minuten von einer Kollegin aufgerufen wird.

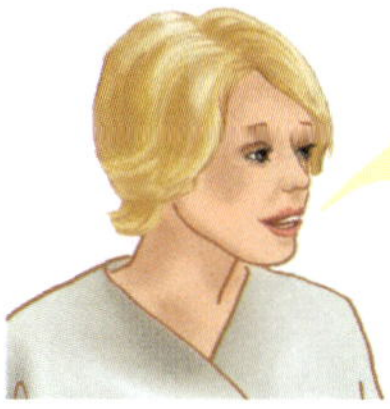

Eine weitere MFA ruft die Patientin auf und sagt ihr, dass sie ihr zum Untersuchungsraum folgen soll.

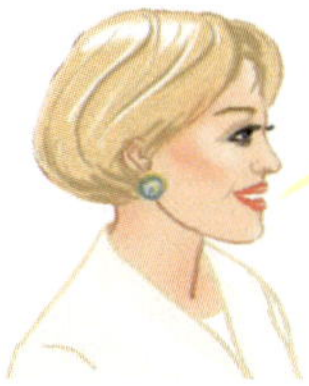

MFA Nr.2 bittet Patientin auf dem großen schwarzen Stuhl Platz zu nehmen.

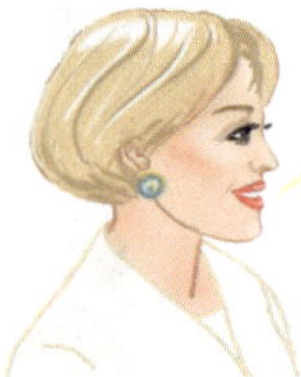

……………………………………………………………………………………………………

……………………………………………………………………………………………………

Die Patientin setzt sich.

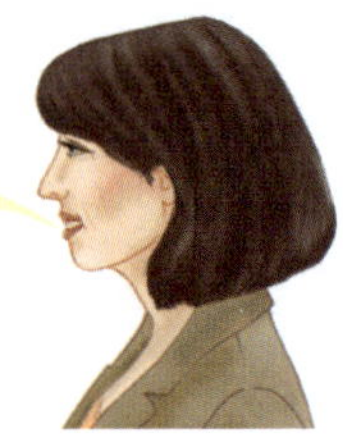

……………………………………………………………………………………………………

MFA fragt die Patientin, ob sie schon einmal einen Hörtest gemacht hat.

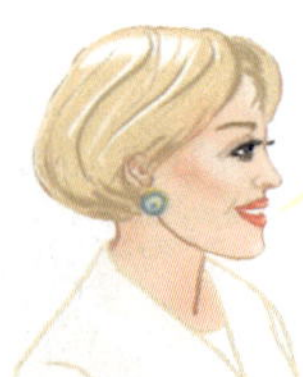

……………………………………………………………………………………………………

……………………………………………………………………………………………………

Die Patientin teilt der MFA mit, dass sie so was noch nie gemacht hat.

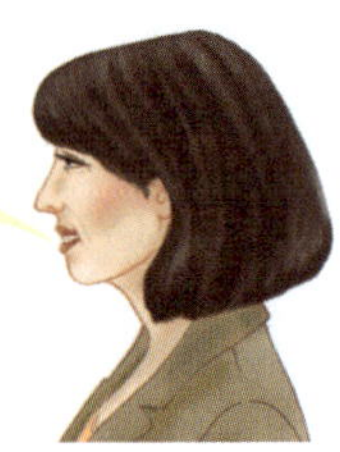

……………………………………………………………………………………………………

MFA erläutert der Patientin, wie der Hörtest abläuft: Die Patientin bekommt einen Knopf zum Drücken und Kopfhörer, die sie aufsetzen soll. Den Knopf soll sie drücken, sobald sie etwas hört. Dann wird die Lautstärke allmählich reduziert, bis die Patientin nichts mehr hören kann. Die Patientin soll wieder durch Knopfdruck anzeigen, wenn sie etwas hört.
Der Test beginnt am rechten Ohr. MFA fragt, ob die Patientin noch Fragen hat.

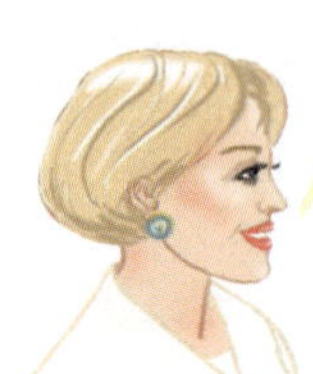

……………………………………………………………………………………………………

……………………………………………………………………………………………………

……………………………………………………………………………………………………

……………………………………………………………………………………………………

……………………………………………………………………………………………………

……………………………………………………………………………………………………

……………………………………………………………………………………………………

Die Patientin hat keine Fragen und ist bereit.

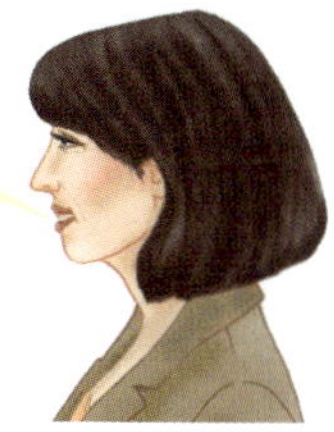

....

MFA teilt der Patientin mit, dass nach dem rechten das linke Ohr getestet wird. Anschließend folgt noch ein zweiter Test.

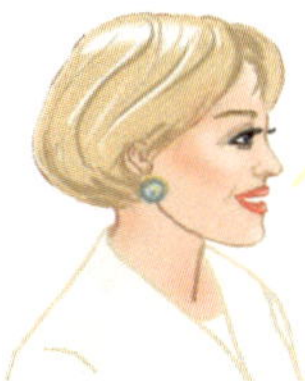

....

....

....

After the first part of the test is completed...

MFA teilt mit, dass jetzt der zweite Test beginnt. Die Patientin bekommt ein Stirnband mit einem Rechteck, das hinter das Ohr kommt und Vibrationen über die Schädelknochen ans Innenohr leitet. Die MFA bittet die Patientin, sich aufs rechte Ohr zu konzentrieren und wieder den Knopf zu drücken, sobald sie rechts etwas hört. Nach dem Messen des rechten Ohres folgt das linke.

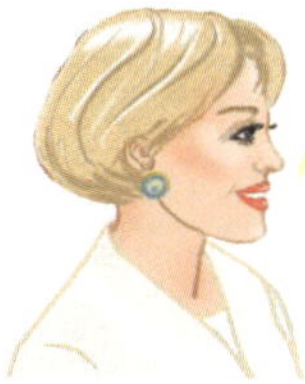

....

....

....

....

....

....

....

Die Patientin signalisiert, dass sie die MFA verstanden hat und bereit ist.

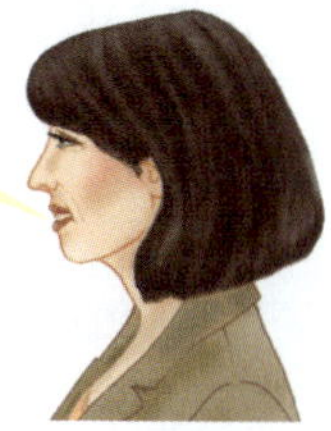

....

MFA teilt der Patientin mit, dass sie jetzt fertig sind und die Patientin noch kurz im Wartezimmer Platz nehmen soll.

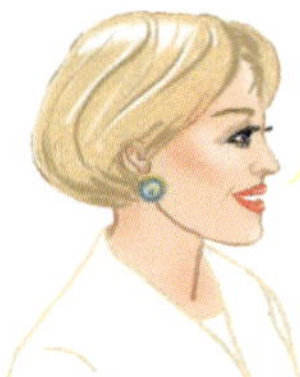

Die Patientin möchte wissen, wie der Hörtest ausgefallen ist.

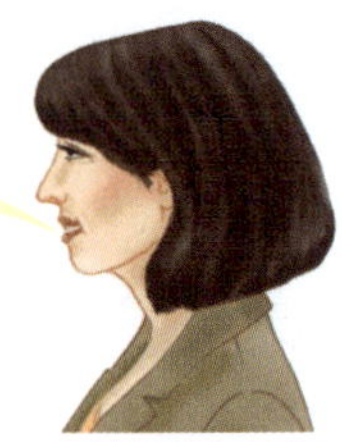

MFA sagt der Patientin, dass der Arzt sich mit ihr über das Ergebnis unterhalten wird....

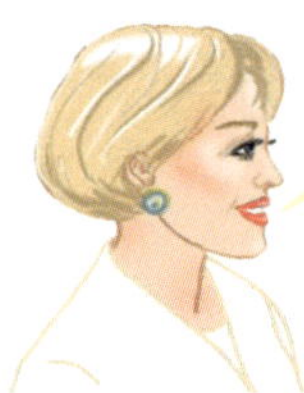

Die Patientin bedankt sich bei der MFA.

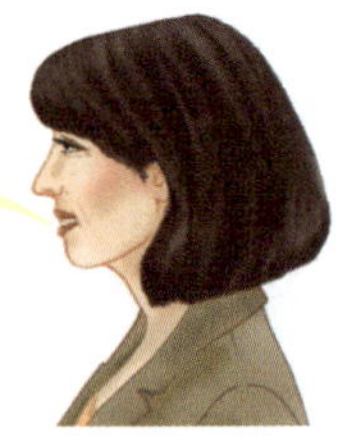

MFA antwortet.

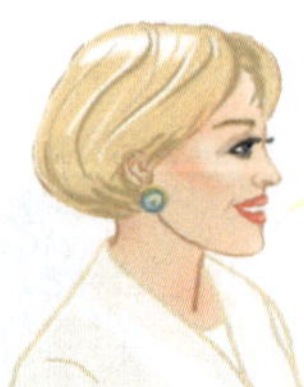

Audiometry WORD SEARCH

5 **Can you find 23 hidden words? Find the hidden message in the remaining letters:**

Y	L	F	O	F	L	B	D	D	V	U	S	D	E	D
M	P	U	O	L	R	R	U	I	E	S	S	N	H	A
R	I	A	U	O	O	E	B	T	O	E	T	A	E	I
S	A	K	R	C	R	R	Q	L	T	S	P	B	A	D
E	S	E	E	E	A	P	G	U	P	O	E	D	R	E
P	H	R	R	T	H	N	D	E	E	M	N	A	I	M
A	C	E	I	E	I	T	C	N	U	N	M	E	N	S
R	A	O	A	R	N	I	H	L	U	Y	C	H	G	I
A	N	C	A	D	A	N	O	C	A	O	I	Y	A	T
T	U	E	S	L	P	V	I	E	E	G	S	H	I	I
E	H	A	I	R	D	H	N	E	H	E	S	S	D	T
L	O	S	A	U	D	I	O	G	R	A	P	H	Y	O
Y	T	F	H	E	A	R	I	N	G	T	E	S	T	H
E	N	O	T	T	S	E	T	D	E	C	I	B	E	L
D	E	A	F	N	E	S	S	E	A	S	R	I	N	G

Hidden message:

Audio Word List

Aussprachehilfe auf CD. Medizinische Fachwörter in den Lesetexten, die nicht in den Audio-Dialogen vorkommen, können hier angehört und die Aussprache geübt werden.

(Track 22, A-C):

A

abdomen
ache
acidity
allergen
amniocentesis
analysis
anaphylactic shock
anemia
anterolateral
antibiotic
anticoagulation
antihistamine
antiserum
applicator stick
artery
asthma
audiogram
audiometry

B

bicarbonate
biopsy
bowel movement
bronchitis
bronchodilator inhaler

C

caecum
capillary
capsule
carbohydrates
carbon dioxide
cardiotocography
cardiovascular disease
catecholamines
chlamydia
cholesterol
circulatory
coagulation
colonoscope
colonoscopy
constipation
contraception
coronary
to cough
creatinine clearance
crutches
cystitis

(Track 23, D-G):

D

decible
deltoid
diabetes
diagnosis
diarrhea
diphtheria
dosage

E

echocardiography
electrode
electrocardiogram
electrocardiography
expiratory

F

fatigue
fecal occult blood test
feces
fibriosis

G

gauze
globules
glucometer
glucose
gynecologist

(Track 24, H-N)

H

haemophilus influenza
hydrochloric acid
hypertension
hyperventilation
hypoglycemia

I

immune system
immunization
to immunize
intestinal examination
intramuscular
irregularity

L

laboratory
lancet
large intestine
laxative
lead apron
leucocytes
ligaments
lung emphysema

M
maneuver
massage
menstruation
microorganism
midstream specimen of urine
muscle

(Track 25, O-R)

O
obstetrics
obstructive disease
oral glucose tolerance test
orthopedic specialist
orthopedist
osteoarthritis
oxygen

P
palpation
palpitation
pediatrician
penicillin
pertussis
peripheral arterial disease
pharmacist
pheochromocytoma
physiotherapy
polyp
preeclampsia
pregnancy
prenatal
prostate
protein
pulmonary
pyelonephritis

R
radiograph
radiography
referral
respiratory
restrictive disease
reversibility testing
rhesus factor

(Track 26, S-W)

S
saline solution
sedative
self-adhering
specimen
spirometer
spirometry
statutory health insurance
sterile
to sterilize
steroid
subcutaneous
suppository
surgery
suture
syndrom

T
tissue
tonsillitis
tourniquet
toxoplasmosis
tranquilizer
transducer

U
ulcer
ulcerative colitis
ureter
urethra
urinary tract
urine
uterine contraction

V, W
vaccine
vaccination
vagina
vertebral column
wheal

Abbreviations (Abkürzungen)

Englische Abkürzungen

GP	general practitioner	Allgemeinmediziner, Hausarzt
MA	medical assistant	Medizinische Fachangestellte
BP	blood pressure	Blutdruck
ABPM	automatic blood pressure measurement	Langzeitblutdruckmessung
ECG	electrocardiography	Elektrokardiogramm (EKG)
COPD	chronic obstructive lung disease	chronisch obstruktive Lungenerkrankungen
FVC	forced vital capacity	Forcierte Vitalkapazität
FEV_1	forced expiratory volume in one second	Einsekundenkapazität
ABG	arterial blood gas (analysis)	Blutgasanalyse (BGA)
pH	measure of acidity	Säuregehalt
UTI	urinary tract infection	Harnwegsinfektion
MSU	midstream specimen of urine	Mittelstrahlurinprobe
HIV	Human immunodeficiency virus	Humanes Immundefizienz-Virus
CTG	cardiotocography (fetal monitoring)	Kardiotokografie
FOBT	fecal occult blood test	fäkaler okkulter Bluttest (Guajak-Test)
OGTT	oral glucose tolerance test	oraler Glukosetoleranz-Test, Zuckerbelastungstest
hrs	hours	Stunden
IgE	immunoglobulin E	Immunglobulin E
ENT	ear nose throat	Hals-Nasen-Ohren

Deutsche Abkürzungen

DAK	Deutsche Angestellten-Krankenkasse
AOK	Allgemeine Orts-Krankenkasse
BEK	Barmer Ersatzkasse
AU	Arbeitsunfähigkeitsbescheinigung
MFA	Medizinische Fachangestellte
BE	Blutentnahme
KHK	Koronare Herzkrankheit
KVK	Krankenversicherungskarte
LZ-RR	LangzeitBlutdruck
EKG	Elektrokardiogramm
mm Hg	Maßeinheit für Druck (Millimeter Quecksilbersäule)
mg/dl	Milligramm pro Deziliter

Word List A–Z

24-hour period innerhalb 24 Stunden
24-hours urine specimen Sammelurin

A

abdomen Bauch, Unterleib
abdominal wall Bauchdecke
abnormal (von der Norm) abweichend
abnormality Unregelmäßigkeit, Missbildung
abrasion Schürfwunde
absorbed aufgenommen
absorbent aufsaugend, saugfähig
absorption Aufnahme, Absorption
accompany (to) begleiten
achieve (to) erreichen
acid-base balance Säure-Basen-Haushalt
acidity Säuregehalt
activity Leistung, Aktivität
additional zusätzlich
adhesive haftend, klebend
adult Erwachsener
advice Rat
advisable empfehlenswert, ratsam
affect (to) auswirken, schädigen
affected betroffen
age Alter
aim Zweck, Absicht, Ziel
airway Luftröhre
alcohol Alkohol
all year long das ganze Jahr über
allergens Allergene
allergic reaction allergische Reaktion
allergist Allergologe
allergy Allergie
allergy testing Allergietest
allowed (to be) dürfen
amniocentesis Fruchtwasseruntersuchung
amount Menge
amplify (to) verstärken
analyze (to) analysieren, auswerten
anaphylactic shock anaphylaktischer Schock
anemia Anämie, Blutarmut
animal hair Tierhaare
ankle Knöchel
antero vordere/r/s
anti-allergic antiallergisch
antibiotics Antibiotika
antibodies Antikörper
anticoagulant Gerinnungshemmer
anticoagulation Gerinnungshemmung
antihistamine Antihistaminikum
anus Anus
applicator stick Applikator
apply (to) gelten (für), zutreffen (auf); auch: anlegen, auftragen
appointment Termin
appointment book Terminbuch
appointment slip Terminzettel
arrange (to) anordnen, durchführen
arterial arteriell
arterial blood arterielles Blut
artery Arterie
asthma Asthma
at least mindestens
attach (to) befestigen, anstecken
audiogram Audiogramm
audiometry Audiometrie
automatic blood pressure measurement (ABPM) Langzeitblutdruckmessung
avoid (to) vermeiden

B

back Rücken
back pain Rückenschmerzen
bacteria Bakterien
band-aid (US) Pflaster
bandage Verband
bandage (to) bandagieren
bandage scissors Verbandsschere
bathroom Toilette, Bad
bean Bohne
bear (to) tragen
beep Piepston
belt Gürtel
bicarbonate Bicarbonat
bill Rechnung
bind (to) binden
biopsy Gewebeentnahme, Biopsie
birth Geburt
birth defect Geburtsfehler
bite Biss
bladder Blase
bladder inflammation Blasenentzündung

blade Klinge, Messer
blanket Decke
bleeding Blutung
bloated aufgebläht
bloating Aufgeblähtsein
block (to) blockieren
blood Blut
blood cells Blutkörperchen
blood creatinine level Kreatiningehalt
blood fats Blutfette
blood flow Blutfluss, Durchblutung
blood gas analysis Blutgasanalyse
blood glucose concentration Blutzuckergehalt
blood pressure Blutdruck
blood sample Blutprobe
blood test Blutuntersuchung
blood type Blutgruppe
body fluid Körperflüssigkeit
body part Körperteil
bodyweight Körpergewicht
bold print fettgedruckt
bone Knochen
bonus booklet Bonusheft
booster Auffrischungsimpfung
boss Chef (umgangssprachlich)
bowel movement Stuhlgang
bra BH
brand name Firmenname
breast Brust
breastfeeding Stillen
breath Atem
breathing Atmung
breathing problems Atemprobleme
bridge (dental bridge) Brücke
bronchitis Bronchitis
bronchodilator Bronchodilator
bruise (to) Blutergüsse bekommen
bruised mit Blutergüssen
bumpy uneben
burning brennend
busy beschäftigt, betriebsam

C

caecum Blinddarm
calcium Kalzium
calculation Ermittlung, Berechnung
cancer Krebs
cancer check-up Krebsvorsorge
capillary Haargefäß
capsules Kapseln
captured eingefangen
carbohydrates Kohlenhydrate
carbon dioxide Kohlenstoffdioxid
cardiotocography (CTG) Kardiotokografie, Wehen- / fetale Herzton-Aufzeichnung
cardiovascular Herz-Kreislauf-, kardiovaskulär
carry (to) beinhalten, tragen
catch (to) auffangen, einfangen
catch up (to) nachholen
catecholomines Katecholamine
cause Grund, Ursache
cause (to) verursachen
caution Vorsicht, Umsicht
cell Zelle
cereals Frühstücksflocken, Müsli
certain bestimmt
certificate Bescheinigung
cervical vertebrae Halswirbelsäule
changing room Umkleidekabine
channel Kanal
charge Gebühr
chest Brustkorb
chest pain Schmerzen in der Brust
chickenpox Windpocken
child health record Kinderuntersuchungsheft
childbirth Entbindung, Geburt
chills Schüttelfrost
chip card Chipkarte
chlamydia Chlamydien
cholesterol Cholesterin
choose (to) wählen
chronic obstructive lung disease (COPD) chronisch obstruktive Lungenerkrankungen
circulatory Kreislauf-
cleansing wipes Reinigungstücher
clench a fist (to) eine Faust machen
cloudy trüb, wolkig
co-insured mitversichert
co-payment Zuzahlung
coagulation Gerinnung
collapse (to) kollabieren, zusammenbrechen
collect (to) sammeln
colon Dickdarm, Kolon-
colonoscopy Darmspiegelung, Koloskopie
come to a conclusion (to) zu dem Ergebnis kommen
common weitverbreitet, häufig vorkommend
company Firma, Unternehmen
complete (to) vollenden
comprehension Verständnis

comprehensive examination umfangreiche Untersuchung
compression Druck, Kompression
compulsory verpflichtend
condition Leiden, Zustand
condom Kondom
confirmed bestätigt
confused verwirrt
connect (to) anschließen
consider (to) beachten
constant andauernd
consult (to) befragen, konsultieren
consultation Sprechstunde, Beratungsgespräch
consulting hours Sprechstunde, Sprechzeiten
consulting room Sprechzimmer
contain (to) beinhalten
container Sammelbehälter
contamination Verunreinigung, Kontamination
contraception Verhütung
contraceptive pill Antibabypille
contract (to) (sich) zusammenziehen
contribution Beitrag, Abgabe
cooperation Zusammenarbeit
COPD (chronic obstructive pulmonary lung disease) chronisch obstruktive Lungenerkrankung
coronary Herz-
coronary heart disease koronare Herzerkrankung
correct richtig
corridor Gang, Flur
costs Kosten
cotton Baumwolle
cotton swab Tupfer
couch Liege
cough (to) husten
course of antiobitics Antibiotika-Kur
cover Umschlag, Deckel
cover (to) abdecken
covered abgedeckt
cracking Knacken
cramps Krämpfe
cranberry juice Cranberrysaft
creamy cremig
creatinine Kreatinin
creatinine clearance Kreatinin-Clearance
Crohn's disease Morbus Crohn
crown (dental crown) Krone
crutches Unterarmgehhilfe, Krücken
cuff Blutdruckmanschette
cure Heilung
cure (to) heilen
current derzeitig, momentan
cut Schnitt
cut (to) schneiden
cycle (to) Rad fahren
cystitis Blasenentzündung, Zystitis

D

dairy products Milchprodukte
damage Schaden
damaged beschädigt
data Daten
deafness Taubheit
decibel Dezibel
decide (to) beschließen
decrease (to) sinken, abfallen
degree Grad, Stufe
deltoid muscle Deltamuskel
dens dicht
density Dichte
dental Zahn-
dental check-up Kontrolluntersuchung der Zähne
dentures Zahnprothese
depend on (to) abhängen von
dermatology Dermatologie
destroy (to) zerstören
detect (to) feststellen, entdecken, auffinden
detection Erkennung, Feststellung
detergent Reinigungsmittel
develop (to) entwickeln
device Gerät
diabetes Diabetes
diagnosis Diagnose
diagnostic test Diagnosetest
diarrhea Durchfall
diet Ernährung
difficulty Schwierigkeit
diphtheria Diphtherie
dirt Schmutz, Dreck
disappear (to) verschwinden, wegfallen
discomfort Schmerz, Beschwerden, Unbehagen
discuss (to) besprechen
disease Erkrankung, Krankheit
disinfect (to) desinfizieren
disinfectant Desinfektionsmittel
disorder Störung, Funktionsstörung
disposiable Einweg-, zum Wegwerfen
dissolve (to) auflösen
distracting ablenkend
distress Gefahr, Not

dizziness Schwindel (Kreislaufproblem)
dizzy schwindelig
doctor's certificate ärztliche Bescheinigung
doctor's practice (US) / surgery (GB) Arztpraxis
dosage Dosierung
dose Dosis
dressing Verband
drops Tropfen
drowsiness Benommenheit
drowsy benommen
drug (US), medicine (GB) Medikament, Medizin, Arznei, Droge
dust mite Staubmilbe

E

earlobe Ohrläppchen
early stage Frühstadium
earrings Ohrringe
ease (to) erleichtern, verringern
ECG stress test Belastungs-EKG
effective wirksam, erfolgreich
effectiveness Wirksamkeit
effervescent tablet Brausetablette
elastic bandage elastische Binde
elbow Ellbogen
electrical shock Stromschlag
electricity Elektrizität
electrocardiogram (ECG) Elektrokardiogram (EKG)
electrocardiography Elektrokardiographie
electrode Elektrode
elevate (to) hoch lagern
elevation Hochlagern
emergency Notfall
emit (to) aussenden, ausstrahlen
emotional stress psychische Belastung
employee Arbeitnehmer
employer Arbeitgeber
empty (to) entleeren
enlarged vergrößert
ENT specialist Hals-Nasen-Ohrenarzt
enter (to) eingeben, eintragen
entrance Eingang
equipment Gerät(e)
escape (to) entweichen
even gleichmäßig
examination Untersuchung
examination table Untersuchungstisch
examine (to) untersuchen
excercise (to) Sport treiben
exempt ausgenommen
exercise ECG Belastungs-EKG
exhale (to) ausatmen
expected voraussichtlich, erwartet
expense Auslagen, Ausgaben
experience (to) wahrnehmen, erleben
exposure Belichten, Bestrahlen
external außen liegend
extremities Gliedmaßen

F

falsify (to) verfälschen
familiar vertraut, bekannt
family doctor Hausarzt
fast (to) fasten, nüchtern bleiben
fasten (to) befestigen, anlegen
fasting blood glucose Nüchtern-Blutzucker
fatal tödlich
fatigue Erschöpfung
fecal fäkal
fecal occult blood test (FOBT) fäkaler okkulter Bluttest
Federal Employment Office Arbeitsamt, Bundesagentur für Arbeit
feel faint (to) eine Kreislaufstörung haben
female weiblich
fetal fötal
fetal growth Wachstum, Entwicklung des Fötus
fever Fieber
fibrosis Fibrose
fit (to) passen
flex (to) biegen
fluids Flüssigkeit
flush (to) spühlen
foot Fuß
forcefully kräftig, heftig
forearm Unterarm
foreign body Fremdkörper
foreskin Vorhaut
form Formular
fracture Bruch, Knochenbruch
free of charge kostenfrei
frequent(ly) häufig
fridge kühlschrank
furthermore außerdem, darüber hinaus

G

gain (to) zunehmen
gap Spalt, Lücke
garage Autowerkstatt
gas bubbles Luftblasen

gauze bandage Mullbinde
gauze pad Zellstoff-Tupfer, Gaze-Kompresse
gel Gel
general practitioner (GP) Allgemeinmediziner, Hausarzt
genital genital, Genital-
gentle sanft
Germany Deutschland
germs Bakterien, Keime
get dressed (to) sich anziehen
get rid of (to) etw. loswerden
get well! gute Besserung!
glasses Brille
globules Globuli
gloves Handschuhe
glucometer Glukometer
glucose Glukose,
glucose level Blutzuckerspiegel, Blutglukosespiegel
glucose test strip Blutzucker-Teststreifen
grandparents Großeltern
guideline Richtlinie
gym Fitnessstudio
gynecologist Gynäkologe, Gynäkologin

H

habit Gewohnheit, Angewohnheit
halfway halb
hall Gang
hand in (to) einreichen, abgeben
hardness of hearing Hörschwierigkeit
harmful gesundheitsschädlich
harmless harmlos
head Kopf
headache Kopfschmerzen
headband Stirnband
heal (to) heilen
healing progress Heilungsprozess
health insurance Krankenversicherung
health insurance card Versicherungskarte
health insurance company Krankenversicherungsgesellschaft
health insurance policy Krankenversicherung
health insurance system Krankenversicherungssystem
healthcare Gesundheitswesen
healthy gesund
hearing aid Hörgerät
hearing impairment Hörbeeinträchtigung
hearing loss Hörverlust
hearing potential Hörpotenzial
heart attack Herzinfarkt
heart muscle Herzmuskel
heart rate Herzfrequenz
heart rhythm Herzrhythmus
heartbeat Herzschlag
heat Hitze
heating pad Heizkissen
heel Ferse
height Größe
hepatitis B Hepatitis B
herbal tea Kräutertee
hesitate (to) zögern
hidden versteckt
high blood pressure Bluthochdruck
hip Hüfte
hollow hohl
hurt (to) schmerzen, weh tun
husband Ehemann
hydrochloric acid Salzsäure
hypertension Bluthochdruck
hyperventilation beschleunigte Atmung
hypoglycemia Unterzucker

I

ice Eis
icepack Eispack
IgE antibodies IgE-Antikörper
ill, sick krank
illness Krankheit
immediate sofort, sofortig
immune system Immunsystem
immunization Impfung
impaired glucose tolerance verminderte Glukosetoleranz
important wichtig
impuls Impuls
inaccurate fehlerhaft, ungenau
include (to) beinhalten
income Einkommen
increase Anstieg, Zunahme
increase (to) verstärken, erhöhen, steigern
increased erhöht
index finger Zeigefinger
indication Indikation, Symptom
infant Säugling, Kleinkind
infected infiziert, angesteckt
infection Infektion
inflammation Entzündung
inflate (to) aufpumpen
influenza Grippe
inform (to) informieren

inhale (to) einatmen
inhaler Inhalator
injection site Injektionsstelle, Einstichstelle
injury Verletzung
insert (to) einführen, einschieben
inspect (to) untersuchen, ansehen
inspiration Einatmung, Inhalation
instruction Anleitung, Anweisung
insulin resistance Insulinresistenz
insulin secretion Insulinsekretion
insurance Versicherung
insurance contribution Versicherungsbeitrag
insurance number Versicherungsnummer
interact (to) zusammenwirken
interaction Wechselwirkung
intercourse Geschlechtsverkehr
interfere (to) Auswirkungen haben auf
internist Internist, Facharzt für innere Krankheiten
intestines Eingeweide
irregular unregelmäßig
irregularity Abweichung, Unregelmäßigkeit
IT company IT-Firma
itchy juckend

J

jam jar Marmeladenglas
jewelry Schmuck
joint Gelenk

K

kidney Niere, Nieren-
knee Knie
knot Knoten

L

lab Labor (Kurzform)
labia Schamlippen
labor pains Geburtswehen
laboratory Labor
lancet Lanzette
lancing device Stechhilfe
large intestine Dickdarm
lateral äußere/r/s
laxative Abführmittel
layers Lagen
lead apron Bleischürze
leucocytes Leukozyten, weiße Blutkörperchen
level Spiegel
ligaments Bänder
likelihood Wahrscheinlichkeit
limit Limit, Grenze
limit (to) begrenzen
line Linie
lining Schleimhaut
liquid flüssig
local örtlich
long term effect Langzeitwirkung
look Aussehen
loose locker
loosen (to) lockern
lumbago Lumbago („Hexenschuss")
lung disease Lungenkrankheit
lung emphysema Lungenemphysem
lung tissue Lungengewebe
lymph node Lymphknoten

M

massage Massage
match (to) abgleichen
maternal mütterlicherseits
maternity record book Mutterpass
measles Masern
measure (to) messen
measurement Messung
medical assistant Medizinische Fachangestellte
medical history medizinische Vorgeschichte, Anamnese
medication Medikation, medikamentöse Behandlung
medicine (GB), drug (US) Medikament, Medizin, Arznei
menstrual cycle Menstruationszyklus
menstruation Menstruation
metabolic Stoffwechsel-, auf den Stoffwechsel bezogen
metabolism Stoffwechsel
microorganism Mikroorganismen
middle finger Mittelfinger
midstream sample (kurz für:) Mittelstrahlurinprobe
midstream specimen of urine (MSU) Mittelstrahlurin-probe
midstream urine Mittelstrahlurin
minimal geringste, geringster, geringstes
minimize (to) verringern
minors Minderjährige
moist feucht
monitor (to) überwachen
monthly monatlich

mosquito bite Mückenstich
motivate (to) motivieren
mouthpiece Mundstück
move (to) bewegen
muesli Müsli
multiple mehrere
muscle Muskel
muscle spasm Muskelkrampf

N

narrow eng
narrowing Verengung
nausea Übelkeit
necessary notwendig
neck Hals, Genick
necklace Halskette
needle Nadel
nerve Nerv
neutralize (to) sich gegenseitig aufheben, neutralisieren

O

observe (to) beobachten
obstetrics Geburtshilfe
obstructive diseases chronisch obstruktive Lungenerkrankungen
obtain (to) erhalten, gewinnen
occur (to) auftreten, vorkommen
offer (to) anbieten
ointment Wundsalbe, Heilsalbe
oral oral-, zum Einnehmen
oral glucose tolerance test (OGTT) oraler Glukosetoleranztest
organ Organ
orthopedic specialist Orthopäde
orthopedist Orthopäde
osteoarthritis Arthrose
otitis media Mittelohrentzündung
over-the-counter frei verkäuflich
overnight über Nacht
overreact (to) überreagieren
overweight (to be) übergewichtig sein
oxygen Sauerstoff
oxygen supply Sauerstoffversorgung

P

pace Geschwindigkeit
pack Packung
pad Kompresse
pain Schmerz, Beschwerden
painkiller Schmerzmittel
painless schmerzlos
pair of tweezers Pinzette
palpation Tastuntersuchung
palpitation Herzklopfen, Herzrasen
pancreas Bauchspeicheldrüse
partial teilweise, Teil-
pass through (to) durchdringen
pass urine (to) Wasser lassen, urinieren
pass wind (to) Blähungen haben, pupsen (ugs.)
pathologic germs pathologische Keime
patient Patient / Patientin
patient (to be) geduldig sein
patient leaflet Beipackzettel
patient's medical history Patientenvorgeschichte
pattern Muster
pea Erbse
pea size erbsengroß
pedal (to) (in die Pedale) treten, Rad fahren
pediatrician Kinderarzt, Kinderärztin
pee (to) (umgangssprachlich für) urinieren
pelvic exam(ination) gynäkologische Untersuchung
penicillin Penizillin
pepper Paprika
percentage Prozent, Verhältnis
perform (to) machen, durchführen
perfumed parfümiert
peripheral arterial disease periphere Arterienerkrankung
persistent anhaltend
personal data persönliche Daten
perspective Blickwinkel
pertussis Keuchhusten
pharmacist Apotheker, Apothekerin
pharmacy Apotheke
pheochromocytoma Phäochromzytom
physical examination körperliche Untersuchung
physically körperlich
physician Arzt, Doktor
physiotherapy Krankengymnastik
pinch Zwicken
place (to) anbringen
plastic bag Plastiktüte
poison Gift

Poland Polen
pollen Pollen
polyp Polyp
potential potenziell, möglich
practice (to) (aus-)üben, praktizieren
preeclampsia Präeklampsie
prefer (to) bevorzugen
pregnancy Schwangerschaft
pregnant schwanger
prenatal care Schwangerenvorsorgeuntersuchung
prepare (to) (sich) vorbereiten
preparing vorbereiten
prescribe (to) verschreiben
prescription Rezept
prescription charge Rezeptgebühr
prescription medication / medicine rezeptpflichtige(s) Medikament(e)
present (to) (vor)zeigen
press (to) pressen
pressure (dressing) Kompresse
pressure bandage Druckverband
preterm labor vorzeitige Wehen
prevent (to) vermeiden, verhindern
preventive health check-up Vorsorgeuntersuchung
previous vorhergehend, früher
prick Pieks
prick (to) stechen, pieksen
prickling sensation Kribbeln
print (to) (aus-)drucken
private health insurance private Krankenversicherung
private insurance Privatversicherung
private prescription Privatrezept
procedure Ablauf, Durchführung
properly genau, richtig
prostate Prostata
prostate gland Vorsteherdrüse
protect (to) schützen
protection Schonung, Schutz
protective screen Schutzscheibe
protein Eiweiß
provided bereitgestellt
pull (to) ziehen
pulmonary function test Lungenfunktionsdiagnostik
pulse rate Pulsfrequenz
pulses Hülsenfrüchte
pump up (to) aufpumpen
puncture Einstich
puncture site Einstichstelle
pyelonephritis Nierenbecken- und Nierenentzündung

Q

quarter Quartal
quit (to) aufhören, aufgeben

R

radiation Strahlung
radiograph Röntgenbild
radiography Röntgenaufnahme
radish Rettich
raise (to) erhöhen
range Bandbreite
rapid rasch, schnell
rare selten
raw roh
reach (to) erreichen
reassure (to) beruhigen
receipt Quittung
receive (to) erhalten
recent vor Kurzem
reception Empfang
recommend (to) empfehlen
record Dokument, Aufzeichnung
record (to) erfassen, festhalten, aufzeichnen, aufnehmen
recording Aufnahme
recover (to) (sich) erholen
rectal rektal, Enddarm-
rectangle Rechteck
rectum Rektum, Enddarm
red blood cells rote Blutkörperchen
redness Rötung
reduce (to) reduzieren, verringern
reduced vermindert
refer (to) überweisen
referral (ärztliche) Überweisung, (auch: Kurzform für Überweisungsschein)
referral note Überweisungsschein
refresh (to) (sich) frisch machen
refrigerated gekühlt
regularly regelmäßig
relative Verwandte, Verwandter
relax (to) entspannen
relevant wichtig
relieve (to) lindern
removal Entfernung
remove (to) entfernen
reoccur (to) wieder geschehen, wieder auftreten
repeat (to) wiederholen
repeated wiederholt

resistant resistent, widerstandsfähig
respiratory Atmungs-
respiratory tract infection Atemwegsinfektion
responsibilty Verantwortung, Verantwortlichkeit
responsible verantwortlich
rest Ruhe
rest (to) ruhen lassen, ausruhen
resting ECG Ruhe-EKG
restricitve diseases restriktive Atemwegserkrankungen
result Ergebnis
reversibility testing Bronchospasmolysetest
Rhesus factor Rhesusfaktor, Rh-Faktor
right angle rechter Winkel
right hand side rechts
ring finger Ringfinger
risk Risko
risk factor Risikofaktor
roll up (to) hoch rollen
routine Routine
routinely routinemäßig
rubella Röteln
run a test (to) einen Test durchführen
running Laufen, Rennen
runny laufend
rupture (to) reißen

S

saline solution Kochsalzlösung
sample Probe
sanitary napkins Monatsbinde
saturation Sättigung
scalpel Skalpell
scar tissue Narbengewebe
scarlet fever Scharlach
scarring Narbenbildung
scratch (to) kratzen
scratch test Ritztest
screen (to) untersuchen, screenen
screening (Vorsorge-)untersuchung
sedative Beruhigungsmittel, Narkosemittel
self-adhering selbsthaftend
self-examination Selbstuntersuchung
sensation Gefühl, Eindruck
sensible sinnvoll, vernünftig
sensitive empfindlich
sensor Sensor
severe schwerwiegend
severity Schweregrad
sex Geschlecht, Geschlechtsverkehr
sexually transmitted diseases sexuell übertragbare Krankheiten
shades of gray Grautöne
shadow Schatten
shape Form
shave (to) rasieren
short-of-breath, shortness of breath außer Atem, Kurzatmigkeit
sick note Krankschreibung
sign (to) unterschreiben
single mother alleinerziehende Mutter
sink Waschbecken
site Stelle
size Größe
skin Haut
skin prick test Pricktest
skin puncture Einstich in die Haut, Hautpunktion
skin rash Hautausschlag
sleepy müde, schläfrig
sleeve Ärmel
small finger kleiner Finger
smear (to) schmieren
smear test Abstrich
smell Geruch
smoke (to) rauchen
sneezing Niesen
social welfare Sozialhilfe
soil Erde, Schmutz
solution Lösung
sore wund
sound frequency Klangfrequenz
sound-audiometry Klangaudiometrie
sound-proof schalldicht
source Quelle
specialist Facharzt
specialize (to) spezialisieren
specimen Probe
speech therapy Sprechtherapie
spirometry Spirometrie
spouse Ehepartner
sprain Verstauchung
spray Spray
spread Verbreitung
spread (to) verbreiten, (sich) ausbreiten
standard vaccinations / standard immunizations Grundimpfungen
staples Klammern
statutory health insurance gesetzliche Krankenversicherung
sterile steril

sterilize (to) sterilisieren
steroid steroid
stiches Naht
stick (to) anhaften, kleben (bleiben), befestigen
stimulate (to) anregen
stitched genäht
stomach ache Magenschmerzen, Bauchschmerzen
stomach cramps Magenkrämpfe
stool Stuhl
stool sample Stuhlprobe
stool test Stuhltest
store (to) aufbewaren
straight away sofort
stress electrocardiogram Belastungs-EKG
stretch (to) strecken, ausstrecken
strip (to) (sich) ausziehen
substance Stoff, Material
suffer (to) leiden
suggestion Vorschlag
suit (to) passen
suitable passend
superficial oberflächlich
support Halt, Unterstützung
support (to) unterstützen
suppository Zäpfchen
surface Oberfläche
surgery Operation (in GB auch: Arztpraxis)
surgery Arztpraxis (GB), (auch: Chirurgie, Operation)
surround (to) umgeben
suspect (to) vermuten
suture Wundnaht
suture kit Nahtmaterial
swabs Tupfer
swallow (to) schlucken
swelling Schwellung
switch (to) wechseln zu
swollen geschwollen
symptom Symptom, Krankheitszeichen
syphilis Syphilis

T

tablets Tabletten
take (to) s.o. temperature / blood pressure hier: messen (Fieber, Blutdruck...)
take a picture (to) ein Bild aufnehmen
take a shower (to) duschen
take advantage of sth. (to) den Vorteil nutzen
take effect (to) Wirkung zeigen
tampon Tampon
tape Heftpflaster
tape (to) festkleben
teeth Zähne
temporary disability zeitliche Arbeitsunfähigkeit
tend to sth. (to) zu etwas neigen
test result Untersuchungsergebnis
test strip Teststreifen
tetanus immunization booster Tetanus Auffrischungsimpfung
thigh Oberschenkel
thread Faden
throat Hals, Rachen
thump Daumen
tight eng
tights Strumpfhose
tiring ermüdend, anstrengend
tissue Gewebe
tissue fluid Gewebeflüssigkeit
toddler Kleinkind
toe Zeh
tonsillitis Mandelentzündung, Angina
tooth Zahn
tooth pain Zahnschmerzen
tourniquet Stauschlauch
toxin Gift
toxoplasmosis Toxoplasmose
traces Spuren
travel (to) wandern
treadmill Laufband
treat (to) behandeln
treatment Behandlung
treatment couch Behandlungsliege
treatment room Behandlungszimmer, Untersuchungszimmer
treatment table Behandlungstisch
tube Röhre, Kanal
tumor Geschwulst, Tumor
twist (to) umknicken, umbiegen

U

ulcer Geschwür
ulcerative colitis Colitis ulcerosa
ultrasound Ultraschall
unborn ungeboren
uncomplicated unkomliziert
undergo (to) sich (etw.) unterziehen
underpants Slip, Unterhose
unemployed arbeitslos
unhealthy ungesund
unpleasant unangenehm

up-to-date auf dem neusten Stand
upper arm Oberarm
ureters Harnleiter
urethra Harnröhre
urge Drang
urgent dringend, akut
urinalysis Harnuntersuchung
urinary tract Harnapparat, Harnwege
urinary tract infection (UTI) Harnwegsinfektion
urinate (to) urinieren, Wasser lassen
urine Urin
urine cup Urinbecher
urine sample Urinprobe
urine test Urintest
usually normalerweise
uterine contractions Geburtswehen

V

vaccination Impfung
vaccination card Impfausweis
vaccine Impfstoff
vagina Vagina
value Wert
various verschiedene
vein Vene
vertebral column Wirbelsäule
viral Virus-, viral
void (to) (ent-)leeren
volume Volumen
vomiting Erbrechen

W

waiting-room Wartezimmer
waste bin Mülleimer, Abfallbehälter
waste product Abfallprodukt
watch Uhr
wear (to) tragen, anhaben
weight Gewicht
wheal Quaddel
wheezing Keuchen
white blood cells weiße Blutkörperchen, Leukozyten
wife Ehefrau
wine Wein
wipe (to) wischen
wipe off (to) abwischen
wire Kabel
within innerhalb von
womb Gebährmutter
wound Wunde
wound management Wundbehandlung
wrap around (to) (um-)wickeln, (herum-)schlingen
wrist Handgelenk
write out (to) ausschreiben, ausstellen

X

X-ray Röntgenbild
X-ray image Röntgenbild
X-ray machine Röntgenapparat
X-ray record card Röntgenpass
X-rays Röntgenstrahlen